All About Adolescence

All About Adolescence

C. G. D. BROOK
The Middlesex Hospital, London, UK

A Wiley Medical Publication

JOHN WILEY & SONS
Chichester · New York · Brisbane · Toronto · Singapore

Library of Congress Cataloging in Publication Data:

Brook, C. G. D. (Charles Groves Darville)
   All about adolescence.

   (A Wiley medical publication)
   Includes index.
   1. Adolescent medicine. I. Title. II. Series.

RJ550.B76   1985   613'.04233   85-16936

ISBN 0 471 90860 6 (pbk.)

British Library of Congress Cataloging in Publication Data:

Brook, Charles G. D.

   All about adolescence.
   1. Adolescence
   I. Title

   305.2'35   HQ796

ISBN 0 471 90860 6

Printed and bound in Great Britain

Contents

Introduction

Adolescence is defined as the process or condition of growing up, that is the period between childhood and maturity. It encompasses, therefore, not only the physical changes of puberty but also the emotional, psychological and social differences between adults and children. It is a period through which all must pass but about which there is little education available, perhaps because the field is so broad.

In medical terms, adolescents are badly catered for. Their problems fall between the spheres of expertise of paediatricians and of the various specialities of adult medicine. On the whole, because they are a healthy section of the population, there are rather few in trouble at any one time, so there are not only few doctors who specialize in this area but also very few facilities. Populations in hospitals are ageing, and adolescents are far too often asked either to choose between the company of elderly people on an adult ward or the hurly burly of a paediatric ward. Neither is ideal.

Parents of adolescent children often feel very isolated. If they are having problems with their adolescent children, they may well be shy to ask for help and, if they do ask, they may not get an answer. Adolescents themselves may worry about the changes that are going on and need to seek some independent reference.

It is with these groups and with professionals in education

and health in mind that this book has been written to try to provide a simple guide to the various changes of adolescence and an explanation of the more common problems which may be encountered.

In writing this book I have drawn heavily on discussions over the years with many adolescent patients and their parents. Miss Karen Miles has not only prepared the manuscript with great skill but also injected it with some common sense. Finally, my wife as well as Charlotte and Henrietta, my teenage daughters, took the time and trouble to read and make valuable comments on the manuscript. I am very grateful to all these people.

PART I

Growing Up

1

Growth

Growth begins at conception and the nine months spent in the uterus is a time of quite phenomenal increase in size and complexity of the body. By the time a baby is born, its length is about one-third of its adult size and the remaining two-thirds takes about 16 years to achieve. It is hardly surprising, therefore, that what happens before birth is so important to our long-term future. Any adverse circumstances in pregnancy lead to impairment of growth and sometimes of function, which can never be recovered—this is why the study of the growth of a baby before it is born has become so important and why the care of pregnant women is so crucial to the welfare of future generations of children.

After birth, growth in height proceeds very rapidly during the first two or three years of life but its rate falls very rapidly, too, so that a baby grows about 20 cm in the first year of life, about 12 cm in the second and 8 cm in the third. By the age of two years, a person is generally about half his or her adult stature (Figure 1.1). Because this is a period of such rapid growth, things that go wrong during it also have long-term consequences. It is, therefore, important to spot failure of growth during these early years and to deal with it if possible. The causes of such failure are sometimes medical, sometimes emotional, but most frequently due to a generally poor environment: food and love and housing are much more important to growth than the things with which doctors deal.

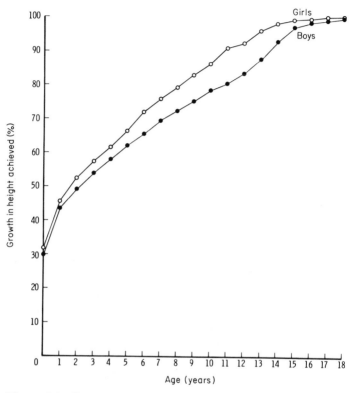

Figure 1.1 Proportions of total height achieved according to age. Note that one-third of height has already been achieved at the end of gestation.

During the primary and junior school years, that is from the ages of three to eleven, growth continues at a fairly steady rate. The rate steadily declines as age advances so that between the ages of three and five the average child grows about 15 cm while between eight and ten the increase is about 10 cm.

Around ten years of age in girls and about two years later in boys, the tempo of growth changes dramatically, for these are the ages when the growth spurts of puberty begin to appear. There is considerable variation in the timing of this growth spurt between individuals. From the onset of puberty to the cessation of growth the average girl gains about 25 cm and a boy about 30 cm. Because boys start from a base height achieved about two years later than that for a girl, the final height of an average man ends up about 12.6 cm (about 5 in) more than that of an average woman. If you, a woman, want to know how tall you would have been had you been born a man, add 12.6 cm (5 in) to your present adult height and if you are a man, subtract this amount to find how tall you would have been as a woman.

These calculations can be used in practice to predict the range of heights which you might expect your children to achieve. For daughters, the final height is likely to be within 8.5 cm (3 1/2 in) either side of the average of the height of the mother and that of the father less 12.6 cm (5 in). The heights of sons have the same range around the mean of the height of the father and the height of the mother with 12.6 cm (5 in) added to it. From such calculations, one can predict earlier in childhood whether the children of given parents are on target in terms of their growth. Please note that adults are very unreliable in their knowledge of their heights and usually overestimate them. Wives and husbands reporting the heights of their spouses are even more unreliable. Parental heights must actually be measured to be of any value in growth assessment.

The average figures conceal enormous individual variation. Thus the range of age for the start of adolescent growth may be between nine and thirteen years in girls and between ten and fifteen years in boys and growth in adolesence may last for as little as eighteen months or for as long as seven years and yet be quite normal. The difference between the rate of growth just before the start of the adolescent growth spurt and the peak of it may be as little as 1 cm per year or as much as 7 cm per year. Thus while mean heights and rates and ages tell us something about human growth in general terms, they are of very little help in individual cases.

GROWTH ASSESSMENT

In order to establish normality of growth and development, it is necessary to compare a child with the heights of his parents and with the heights of his peers. This process is called growth assessment. The first prerequisite is an accurate measurement of the child's height and measurement of the heights of the parents. Using a chart such as that shown in Figure 1.2, a centile chart for height, an idea can be gained of where the child is in relation to his or her peers and whether this is appropriate for the heights of the parents which are entered at their centile positions. At this stage, a doctor will often call for a measurement of skeletal age by an X-ray examination of the hands and wrists in order to make a prediction of final height. This is not a diagnostic manoeuvre, because at this stage one has no idea of whether growth, which is an active process, is normal. It is aimed simply at establishing a target. A single measurement of height and bone age certainly does not consititute any sort of investigation.

Growth is an active process and the rate at which a child is growing is much more important to establish than what he has previously achieved, which is now history and not able to be influenced. In order to tell whether a child is growing normally, two measurements are required separated by a period of time. The length of time between measurements is not critical but it has to be sufficient for the errors in

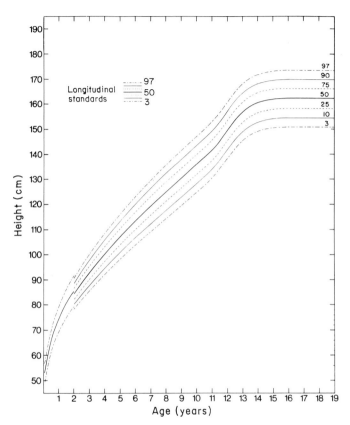

Figure 1.2   Centile height chart for girls. If one stands one hundred normal girls of four years in a line, there will be a height above and below which the stature of fifty of the girls will be found. This height happens to be 100 cm and is the fiftieth centile. Centile lines can be drawn for any number and the centiles shown (3 to 97) have no special significance. Where a child lies on such a chart depends upon many interacting genetic and environmental influences and a single height plot means very little in diagnostic terms. Based on the Tanner-Whitehouse growth and development chart 3A and reproduced by permission of Castlemead Publications.

measuring to be much smaller than the increase in height which would be expected. In all but the most rapidly growing children a minimum of three months is required for this purpose if the equipment for measuring is good and the technique very careful. Even then, considerable caution is needed not to overinterpret a growth rate measured over such a short period of time. In less ideal circumstances, such as at home or in schools, it is not worth measuring children more frequently than at a six month interval. When a measurement of rate has been achieved, it can be compared to a rate chart (Figure 1.3).

BODY PROPORTIONS

Growth of the legs and growth of the spine contribute about equally to total height gains in childhood. When the adolescent growth spurt begins, the feet and the legs start to grow first and increase in rate of growth of the spine begins somewhat later, continuing after growth of the legs has ceased. Thus a boy stops growing out of his trousers (and shoes) before he stops growing out of his jackets.

Other body proportions change during this period and the widening of the shoulders and hips comes towards the very end of the growth of puberty. It must be remembered, however, that overall body shape has much to do with the acquisition of fat and muscle and is not just a consequence of bony development. Fat and muscle have patterns of growth all of their own that are very important to the final appearance of adult men and women.

Nor do changes of shape cease when growth in height comes to its end. There are very obvious differences between the appearance of men and women towards the end of their twenties compared to the end of their teenage years, although these differences are rather poorly documented by

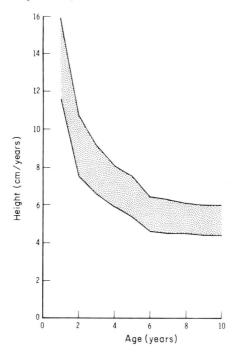

Height velocity: acceptable limits for boys and girls

How to use this chart:

1. Measure height on two occasions.

2. Plot the rate of growth (cm/year) against the age of the child midway between the two measurements.
   e.g. heights measured at ages 4 and 6 show a difference of 12 cm. Rate is 6 cm/year which should be plotted at age 5.

3. Seek advice for rates falling outside the hatched area.

Figure 1.3   Height velocity chart: acceptable limits for boys and girls. Note that measurements of rate of growth are largely independent of sex and of height which has already been achieved.

human biologists. They are of considerable importance to the fashion trade and are a further indication that adolescence covers a period much longer than the time over which the majority of growth and the acquisition of secondary sexual characteristics take place.

GROWTH IN WEIGHT

In a normal adult about 20 per cent of total body weight is accounted for by fat. Because the density of fat is rather less than that of water, the actual amount of fat in terms of volume is rather greater than this, and an increase in weight which is due to obesity is due to a much larger volume of fat accumulated. Of the remaining 80 per cent of body weight, which is called the lean body mass, 72 per cent is water. This water is divided between that which is inside the cells of the body and that which is widely distributed between the cells of the body in direct continuity with the blood stream.

Consideration of these figures will show that the measuring of body weight to assess growth is a poor substitute for measuring height, since only about 10 per cent of weight actually results from the solid elements of the body. Naturally, as height and cellular mass increase, weight does increase, but this is largely due to the increase in total body water. As about 2 litres of water pass in and out of the body each day there are bound to be substantial changes in weight as the day goes on according to the state of input and excretion of food and drink. In practical terms, what this means is that unless growth is proceeding at a very fast rate (as it does in the newborn nursery) weighing a child to assess his growth is likely to mislead because the errors of weighing exceed the increments that might be expected. An average child gaining weight between the ages of two and eight gains about 2 kg *per year*: we have already seen that the daily fluctuations of fluids are about 2 litres (2 kg) *daily*. So much for weight!

GROWTH OF BODY FAT

Body fat is a very peculiar organ. It is crucial to our health and well-being and much abused by the dictates of fashion. We understand very little about what determines its amount save the absolute certainty that a continuous intake of food above what we require for everyday life leads to an increase in total body fat and that a continuous intake of food which is less than metabolic requirements leads to a loss of body fat. There is, however, a substantial variation in the number of calories which different individuals eat and it is remarkable how constant body weight generally remains despite these large variations.

Curiously, in spite of appearances to the contrary, people are extraordinarily self-regulating about what they eat and it is actually very difficult to feed individuals continuously, even under experimental conditions, either more or less than they actually require. Considering the amount that is written about diet, it is remarkable that more people are not fat when it is considered that a continuous daily intake of 10 calories in excess of requirements (1/4 teaspoon of sugar) over the course of a whole year would lead to an excess of fat of about 400 g. It is because of the extraordinary complexity of energy balance that so many freakish ideas and money-spinning projects arise in this field.

Body fat increases rapidly during the first year of life and reaches a peak which is slightly earlier and slightly less in boys than in girls (Figure 1.4). During the period between one and seven years of age there is a gradual decline in skinfold thicknesses in both sexes, although as they are growing at the same time, the total amount of body fat increases. In

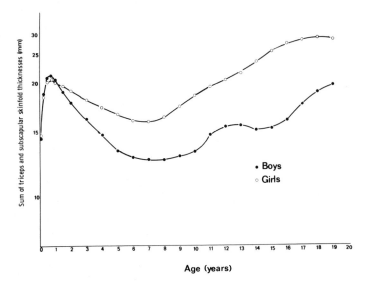

Figure 1.4   Changes in body fat with age.

the middle of childhood there is a small increase in the rate of growth in height, but a marked increase in the thickness of body fat. Exaggeration of this increase, especially in boys, sometimes presents as a problem of clinical obesity, but the prepubertal increase of fat is both very variable and very little understood.

During puberty, fat is acquired by both sexes but the total amount gained is rather greater in women than in men and the distribution of body fat in the two sexes becomes rather different. In children, the thickness of fat over the arms and legs is considerably greater than over the trunk. As puberty approaches, limb fat is gradually shed in both sexes and by the time that the skinfold thicknesses are approximately equal one can predict that the growth spurt in height of adolescence will be under way. As time goes on, the fat is further redistributed and in men limb fat becomes progressively reduced and trunk fat increases. In women the loss of limb fat is less marked and in some cases may not occur, but there is an accumulation of fat around the shoulders and hips.

By the time that puberty is complete there are thus clearly marked differences in the body composition of men and women, especially as men preferentially accumulate muscle mass as a result of the stimulation by male sex hormones. These changes together with those of body proportion which have already been mentioned are really more important to the differences in appearance between adult men and women than are the actual secondary sexual characteristics. They serve also to emphasize the difference between adolescence, which, according to the *Oxford Dictionary*, extends to twenty-five years of age in males and twenty-one years of age in females, and puberty, which may be defined as the acquisition of reproductive capability which is completed at a much younger age.

2

Puberty

FEMALE SEXUAL DEVELOPMENT

About half the population of boys and girls can be expected to show some signs of pubertal development before their twelfth birthday. The earliest signs in a girl are generally seen in breast development and in girls the growth spurt which is associated with puberty begins as soon as breast development starts. Pubic hair generally appears at about the same time but may sometimes precede breast development. A discrepancy of more than one year between the appearance of pubic hair and the appearance of breast development in either direction can be an important indicator of a medical problem.

Breasts and pubic hair and the rate of growth all increase during the next eighteen months or so but menarche (the onset of the monthly periods) does not occur until after the peak of the growth spurt has been passed and certainly not until breast and pubic hair development is well advanced (Figure 2.1). After the first menstrual period has occurred, vaginal bleeding may be far from regular for a number of years. This is due to the fact that the first menstrual periods are not regularly associated with ovulation (the production of mature eggs from the ovary) and until regular ovulatory cycles are established, which takes two years on average and sometimes as long as five years, regular menstrual bleeding will not be found. Contrary to commonly held belief,

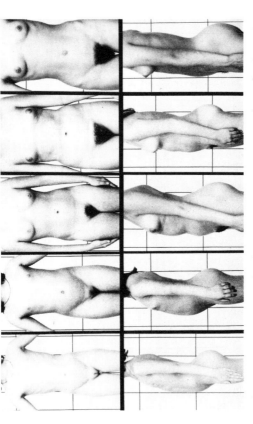

Figure 2.1 Stages of pubertal development in girls. In stage 1 there are no signs of puberty. In stage 2 the breast bud begins to swell and the diameter of the areola enlarges; there is a sparse growth of long, slightly pigmented hair over the labia. By stage 3 the breast and areola have enlarged further but there is no separation of their contours. Pubic hair becomes darker and spreads over the junction of the pelvis. At stage 4 the areola and nipple form a secondary mound above the level of the breast. Pubic hair, which is now adult in type, covers an area smaller than in the adult and does not spread to the thighs. Menarche usually occurs at this stage. The areola at stage 5 becomes continuous with the contour of the breast leaving the nipple to project. Pubic hair is adult in quality and quantity.

growth does not stop as soon as the periods begin: on average growth continues for at least two years, although at an increasingly slow rate, after menarche.

The timing of events of puberty in girls is shown in Figure 2.2. Almost all girls will have shown some sign of pubertal development by their fourteenth birthday. A few will have signs of development before the ninth birthday. Girls whose development starts before or after these ages are probably just at the extremes of normality rather than having anything actually wrong with them, especially those who start early, but parents should not delay in seeking a medical opinion about their daughters whose development falls outside these ages. In particular, it is most important to have an adequate explanation of delayed puberty in a fifteen year old girl and not just to assume that all will be well. In this context it is worth pointing out that, as long as puberty has

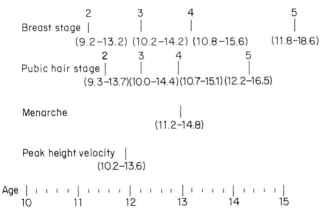

Figure 2.2 Timing of events of puberty in girls. The ages by which 50 per cent of girls have achieved the stage of puberty shown in Figure 2.1 are shown together with the range of age for 3 and 97 per cent of girls to have achieved a particular stage.

started, it is unlikely that it will become arrested, and a doctor can afford to be much more sanguine about a girl aged seventeen years who has not yet seen her periods, as long as all other aspects of her pubertal development (breasts, pubic hair and growth) are normal.

The time that it takes for a girl to go through puberty varies considerably, but 50 per cent of girls will have completed their pubertal development in about three years; 3 per cent may take as short a time as eighteen months but 97 per cent of girls will have completed all the stages of puberty over a period of five years. Advice should be sought for rates of development which are greater or less than these. Advice should also be sought if there is no detectable advance of the stage of puberty over one year. Irregular periods are normal for some years after menarche but if they are persistently irregular for longer than five years, it is worth seeking advice.

MALE SEXUAL DEVELOPMENT

In boys, the earliest signs of puberty are to be seen in the increase in the size of the testes and in changes in the appearance of the penis and scrotum (Figure 2.3). These changes occur at more or less the same ages as breast development begins in girls, that is around the twelfth birthday, but the increase in growth rate occurs much later in the sequence of pubertal development, roughly at a time comparable to menarche in a girl. It is, therefore, no good expecting growth to occur in male puberty until the genitalia and testes are well developed (stage 3/4). Many boys, expecially those with late puberty, are very disappointed at the time that it takes for the pubertal growth spurt to develop. They are often caused unnecessary suffering by false reassurance that they will start to grow as soon as they start to develop. This is not the case.

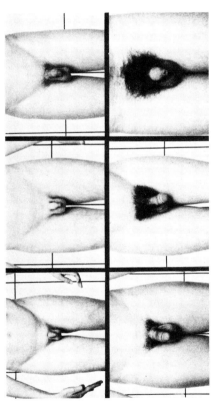

Figure 2.3   Stages of pubertal development in boys. In stage 1 the penis and the testes are small and there is no sign of pubic hair. In stage 2 the testes have begun to enlarge and the skin of the scrotum reddens and changes in texture. There is little growth of the penis at this stage. Pubic hair is long and downy but only slightly pigmented. By stage 3 the testes and scrotum have grown more and the penis begins to enlarge. Darker and coarser hair spreads sparsely over the junction of the pelvis. At stage 4 there is increased size of the penis and development of the glans. The scrotal skin becomes darker and the pubic hair, although adult in quality, covers an area considerably less than that in the adult. Genital and pubic hair development is complete at stage 5. Later pubic hair may spread more widely and is rated as stage 6.

It is largely due to the delay in the onset of the pubertal growth spurt that adult men are taller than adult women. The delay of two years accounts for about 10 cm (4 in) of the difference; boys actually grow at a faster rate than girls when they do start their growth spurt but it is over quicker and they stop growing more quickly than girls so that this part of the growth process accounts only for 2.5 cm (1 in) more difference in final height (see page 5).

Very similar limits apply to the onset of pubertal signs (Figure 2.4) and the duration of puberty in boys as they do in girls. Thus, advice should be sought about a boy whose development begins before the age of nine years and a failure to show any signs of development in puberty by the fourteenth birthday deserves the active consideration of a doctor. In most cases, there are actually signs of development at the age of fourteen, but they may be relatively

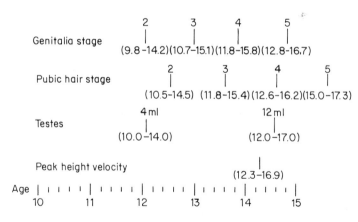

Figure 2.4   Timing of events of puberty in boys. The ages by which 50 per cent of boys have achieved the stage of puberty shown in Figure 2.3 are shown together with the range of age for 3 and 97 per cent of boys to have achieved a particular stage.

difficult to observe since the earliest changes are simply an increase in the size of rather small testes.

Since breast appearance is obvious while testicular enlargement is not and girls start to grow in puberty as soon as their breasts begin to develop whereas boys have to wait for a further eighteen months to start growing quickly, the myth is firmly established that female puberty is significantly advanced in comparison to the events in males. Although this is not actually true, the changing size and appearance of girls at this age entrains a cultural and emotional climate which is extremely important.

Menarche, the onset of menstruation, is one of the latest events to occur in female pubertal development. From the point of view of the mechanisms of normal puberty (see Chapter 3) menarche is not an important event since it is bound to occur if the other changes of puberty are normal. From the point of view of the individual girl and her family, however, it remains an event of signal importance and is generally recognized as being the point of transition from childhood to the status of adult woman. There is no event in male puberty which is so obviously definable and the outward signs of male development, the growth of facial hair and the breaking of the voice, occur much later than the development of reproductive capability. Fifty per cent of boys have broken voices and are shaving by the age of sixteen and 95 per cent will have reached this stage of development by the age of eighteen.

The appearance of breast development in girls, genital development in boys and body hair in both sexes (secondary sexual characteristics) is not synonymous with puberty, which is defined as the attainment of reproductive capability. As has already been indicated, girls are usually not reproductively capable until about one to two years after menarche. On the other hand, spermatogenesis begins in boys as soon as their testes begin to enlarge, and although the finding of spermatozoa in early morning urine is not necessarily equated with the acquisition of fertility, there seems little doubt that by the time a boy is well advanced in puberty and having nocturnal emissions of semen, as well as being able to produce a masturbation specimen containing active sperms, he will be fertile.

While menarche is not synonymous with the attainment of reproductive capability, the changes in the female genital tract which occur during puberty are the direct response to oestrogen secretion and thus precede menarche. The walls of the vagina become soft and pink and the vagina increases in length and may secrete a considerable amount of discharge. There is a general increase in body fat and this occurs also around the vulva (entrance to the vagina) so that it becomes plump and rounded and the skin takes on a relatively wrinkled appearance not unlike the appearance of the scrotum in the male. Thus the potential for sexual intercourse in the female considerably precedes reproductive capability, which is the reverse of what occurs in the adolescent male.

3

Influences on the Growth Process

TIMING

Differences in the timing of growth and development, especially adolescent development, make a substantial contribution to the differences between children within a culture. In terms of stature, children of the same age attending the same school may differ by as much as 20 cm, and the tallest and smallest children have a very different outlook on life which may not only impinge on their relationships with their peers and relatives but also on their school performance. Although much of the variation in height may be genetically determined, a considerable amount of it will be due to the fact that early maturing children will generally be taller than late maturing children, even though their final adult heights may not be very different.

What controls timing is obscure. In examining patients with delayed growth, a family history of later maturing is often elicited but just as often it is not and there are no studies which have systematically examined the timing of the events of puberty in suceeding generations. What is needed is for the children of parents who were themselves the subjects of one of the longitudinal growth studies to be followed through their own growth and puberty.

The mechanisms which underlie the timing of the events of growth are poorly understood and we are rather like weather forecasters. We can have a rough idea in any individual cases of more or less what is going to happen from what has happened already, but it is quite difficult at a single moment in time, without other information of a longitudinal nature, to know how fast things will develop.

GENETIC INFLUENCES

While racial differences play an obvious part in determining the variation of human growth (and standards are available from many countries), the differences between populations in terms of growth and development are much smaller than the variations within cultures. Also, while the timing of the major events may be somewhat different, the rate at which they then proceed is fairly common within the human species. Thus while it may be desirable to have appropriate standards for the population with which one is dealing, rates of growth vary little between different populations and international standards may be applied. Rates of growth are also relatively independent of growth which has already taken place.

The genetic influences on body proportions (height, weight, fat and so on) have been fairly extensively researched. About two- thirds of the total variation in height is genetically determined, which is why the heights of parents are well worth recording in the growth assessment of their offspring (page 5). Since weight is largely determined by height, its genetic determination is also important, but the contribution made by genetic influences to weight is less than that made to height because the amount of body fat is not strongly genetically determined.

If one measures skinfold thickness in children and their parents (Figure 3.1), one finds that genetic influences account for only about one-third of the variation. In other words, 70 per cent of the variation in body fatness is attributable to environmental influences. Since families usually share the same common environment, resemblances between them may appear to reflect a genetic pattern when in fact they reflect the common environment. Identical twins resemble each other not only because they look alike but also because they are treated alike, wear the same clothes and so on.

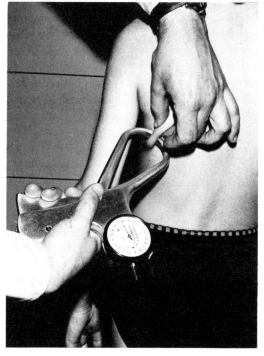

Figure 3.1   Measurement of skinfold thickness as an index of nutritional state.

The genetic influences on the adolescent process are hardly understood at all and, even if they were, they would only be applicable in the most general of ways. It is unwise to take a general principle and apply it to an individual case because of the importance of other (environmental) influences. Just because there is a family history of short stature or late development, it does not mean that a child of such a family cannot have another condition, nor that what was not treated in the parents may not now be treatable. Doctors can now use treatments to alter growth and development which were not available in earlier generations.

ENVIRONMENTAL INFLUENCES

Food is essential for growth in general and for pubertal development in particular. A great deal of discussion has arisen about the influence of nutrition on pubertal development which has been focused in the minds of many doctors on the so-called 'critical weight at menarche' hypothesis. In this theory, it is held that a girl must achieve a specific weight (47 kg) before she will successfully go through puberty.

This is actually a common misunderstanding of the theory and of the ideas of Dr Rose Frisch, whose real message is that successful reproduction demands a certain nutritional standard which may well be individually determinable. Once again, what has happened is that a general principle, which has much to commend it, has been adapted for individual circumstances, which is not a sensible thing to do.

Nevertheless, there are psychiatric disturbances which lead to a restriction of calorie intake (anorexia nervosa) and this is certainly associated with arrest or failure of pubertal development. Undernutrition as a cause of pubertal delay is not all that uncommon and is seen not only in people who have psychological problems but also in children with poorly treated asthma and in diabetic children having problems with their diabetic control (see part III).

Overnutrition also effects growth and development. Increased nutrition during a period of rapid growth appears to increase growth rate but this is compensated by an advance in general maturation. Thus obese (tall) children tend to mature relatively early and to stop growing early, which is why they do no not become tall adults.

EMOTIONAL CLIMATE

It is often difficult to separate the effects of socioeconomic circumstances, which include nutritional influences, from the direct effects of emotional stress. Further, being tall or short or being early or late in maturation considerably influences the emotional development of a child. The complex emotional events which are associated with adolescence are poorly enough understood in normally developing children, and while there is a great deal of talk of psychological influences on physical development, there are very few facts on which to base a meaningful discussion.

Nevertheless, there is no doubt that children starved of affection grow badly and may well grow better if they are removed from an inclement environment. Unhappy children can have very abnormal endocrine function (see below) which recovers in a different environment, so there is no gainsaying the effect of emotional climate on bodily function.

While this applies to childhood generally (and any child who thrives in a hospital environment should be regarded with suspicion), it is especially important in adolescence. For example, I have seen several diabetic children referred for a failure to develop in puberty. Their problem has not generally been the quality of their diabetic control, which is usually the ostensible reason for the referral, but their inability to cope with the pressures of their condition together with the pressures at home, school and with their peer group.When the heat is taken out of the emotional problem, usually without detectable alteration in the quality of diabetic control, puberty has progressed without problem.

The same phenomenon can be observed in the many instances of chronic childhood illness (of which asthma is a notable case in point) and certainly can be induced by any problems of an emotional type, parental divorce being one regrettably common cause. The mechanism is difficult to nail because the mere fact of intervention may be a sufficient alteration of climate to 'unblock' the system.

ENDOCRINE INFLUENCES

All the hormones of the body (the chemical messengers which are transported in the blood stream and control bodily function) are important to the process of growth and development, which is why the monitoring of growth in childhood gives the best overall guide as to whether the body is functioning normally. If it fails in any respect, growth slows and thus a child who is growing normally is unlikely to have a serious problem; poor growth needs urgent explanation, diagnosis and treatment.

While the parathyroid glands, which regulate calcium metabolism, the pancreas, which regulates glucose metabolism, the adrenal medulla, kidney and gut are all extremely important, the hormones which are most directly concerned with normal growth and development are those of the hypothalamo-pituitary-target gland axes (Figure 3.2).

The hypothalamus, which lies right in the centre of the brain, secretes a series of rather small (peptide) hormones

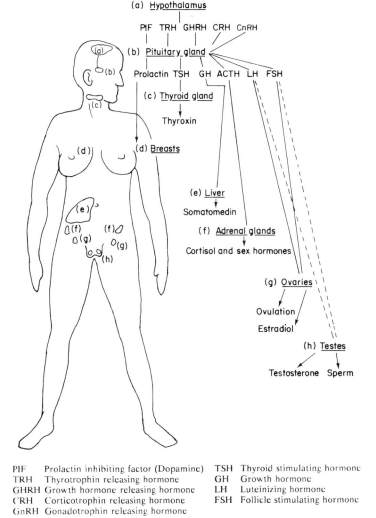

PIF	Prolactin inhibiting factor (Dopamine)	TSH	Thyroid stimulating hormone
TRH	Thyrotrophin releasing hormone	GH	Growth hormone
GHRH	Growth hormone releasing hormone	LH	Luteinizing hormone
CRH	Corticotrophin releasing hormone	FSH	Follicle stimulating hormone
GnRH	Gonadotrophin releasing hormone		

Figure 3.2 The hormones of the hypothalamo-pituitary-target gland axes.

which travel in the pituitary blood supply and influence the release of much larger peptide hormones from the pituitary gland itself. These travel in the general circulation and have their effects on the various endocrine glands in the body. It is the secretion of these endocrine glands which are responsible for normal growth and development.

While the secretions of the thyroid gland (thyroxine) and of the adrenal gland (both cortisol and the sex steroids) play a part in normal adolescent development, for the purposes of this discussion we need to concentrate on growth hormone and on the sex hormones.

Growth Hormone

Growth hormone is a single-chain polypeptide of 191 amino acids. It is required for growth in height, for growth of bone mass and for bone maturation and has complex effects on the metabolism of proteins, carbohydrates and lipids. For the most part it is believed that these actions are achieved by the stimulation of production of growth factors called somatomedins, mainly in the liver.

Growth hormone is synthesized continuously and stored in secretory granules, from which it is released in response to a variety of stimuli. There is a growth hormone releasing hormone which is secreted by the hypothalamus and which is probably secreted continuously in a pulsatile fashion. Another hormone, called somatostatin, acts as an inhibitor of the system and at present we believe that growth hormone release, which occurs in episodes mainly associated with sleep and exercise, occurs when the somatostatin brake is released. Thus, although growth hormone releasing hormone is important for the synthesis of growth hormone, it is probably not intimately connected with its release in normal subjects.

Growth hormone appears in the human foetal pituitary gland about three months after conception. Pituitary growth hormone content increases with foetal age but the role of growth hormone in the foetus remains unknown. At birth the levels of growth are higher in the infant than they are in the mother and they decrease progressively from forty-eight hours of life. From three months of age growth hormone is beginning to be secreted more actively at night than in the daytime, which is the pattern seen during childhood, and the production rate of growth hormone is broadly similar to the rate at which the individual grows. Indeed, it seems probable that the total secretion of growth hormone during childhood is what governs how tall an individual becomes and is possibly the way by which the genetic determination is expressed. It may be possible in the future, therefore, to determine final height by pharmacologically augmenting or decreasing growth hormone secretion.

Hormones Responsible for Sexual Development

The hormones which are most important for pubertal development are those secreted by the testes or ovaries. Testosterone in a boy or estradiol in a girl are secreted as a result of exposure of the testes or ovaries to pituitary gonadotrophin (LH, luteinizing hormone, and FSH, follicle stimulating hormone) secretion. These in turn depend upon secretion by the hypothalamus of gonadotrophin releasing hormone (GnRH).

The hypothalamus secretes gonadotrophin releasing hormone in a pulsatile fashion from around the fifth month of gestation (that is four months before birth) throughout an individual's entire life. This means that the mechanism for sexual maturation is intact long before the changes of puberty actually take place. At present it is not fully understood why the prepubertal child does not usually show signs of sexual maturation until the ages that have previously been discussed. Many theories have been advanced to explain the timing of the onset of puberty, but recent experimental work in patients who have not developed normally in puberty strongly suggests that it is the strength of the gonadotrophin releasing hormone pulse which is most important. This stimulates pituitary gonadotrophin secretion which induces maturation of the testes and ovaries. To what extent the development of the gonads in foetal life depends upon this mechanism is not known.

The probable sequence of events is as follows: pulses of gonadotrophin releasing hormone are secreted every 90 minutes throughout life. During intrauterine life, when the sex hormones of the mother are circulating in the blood of the baby, the testes and the ovaries form. The testes contain the (Leydig or interstitial) cells which produce testosterone (male sex hormone) and the seminiferous tubules which will produce sperm. In foetal life testosterone is responsible for the development of the male external genitalia (the growth of the penis). The seminiferous tubules (actually the sertoli cells) secrete an important hormone in foetal life called antimüllerian hormone. This prevents the development of the uterus and fallopian tubes in a male baby. Without the production of these hormones the baby develops as a female. Thus if there is a failure of gonadal development for any reason, a baby is delivered which is apparently female, according to the appearances of the genitalia and the presence of a uterus. In a normal female foetus, the ovary has no function, but by the time of birth the ovaries contain all the ova that are necessary for a lifetime of reproductive capability and many more in addition, something in the order of one million eggs.

After birth, the strength of the pulses of gonadotrophin

releasing hormone is probably very low and remains so during early childhood. The pulses certainly continue and, using newer techniques of imaging (ultrasound), one can see in girls from the age of two or three years onwards ovarian follicles waxing and waning over longish periods. These follicles produce some female sex hormone (oestradiol) which is important for normal growth. In a child who has no ovaries one can see quite clearly the effect of oestrogen deficiency on growth rate and on bone structure before puberty. We presume that testes behave in the same sort of way in males.

As the years go by, the gonadotrophin releasing hormone pulse becomes stronger, although we do not believe that its frequency alters significantly. As it becomes stronger, the cells of the pituitary gland begin to produce more gonadotrophin in response to the pulses, and puberty is heralded by a marked increase in the pulsatile secretion of luteinizing hormone (LH) which causes the testes to produce testosterone and the ovarian follicles to start to synthesize oestradiol. As puberty progresses, pulsatile FSH secretion occurs, which causes the amount of oestradiol secreted by the ovarian follicles to increase and the testes to get larger in response to growth of the seminiferous tubules. The major physical changes of puberty result from the secretion of testosterone by the testes and oestradiol by the ovaries.

From this description it can be seen that the mechanism of puberty is a gradual increase in the size of the pulses of gonadotrophin releasing hormone, and it is likely that this increase continues during early reproductive life. Certainly, the doses of gonadotrophin releasing hormone which have to be used to treat an adult man or woman to induce fertility are quite a lot larger than those which are needed to treat a child to induce the changes of puberty.

The Menstrual Cycle

As many people believe that menarche is the most important event of female puberty, it is important to understand the events of the menstrual cycle which puts menarche into its proper place in the endocrine events of puberty.

At the start of each menstrual cycle, a crop of ovarian follicles (about 20) begins to mature in response to FSH secreted by the pituitary gland as a result of the pulsatile gonadotrophin releasing hormone secretion mentioned above. These follicles grow and begin to synthesize oestradiol in response to rather small rises in the levels of LH and FSH. FSH is responsible for the actual secretion of oestradiol and the ovarian follicles make receptors to receive the FSH in proportion to how good they are at making oestradiol.

As the levels of oestradiol rise, so there is a feedback mechanism which means that the pituitary gland produces less FSH in response to the same signal from the hypothalamus. This means that only the ovarian follicles which have the most receptors for FSH can continue in oestradiol production. By this very clever mechanism we get to a situation where a single ovarian follicle becomes dominant over all the other follicles which then atrophy and are lost for ever. The remaining single follicle produces enough oestradiol to suppress FSH secretion, but when it too begins to fail because FSH levels fall progressively, it triggers a surge of LH in the mid cycle which brings about ovulation.

After ovulation has occurred, the cells of the follicle which remain form a yellow body called a corpus luteum which secretes progesterone and oestradiol during the second half of the menstrual cycle. Unless the ovum is fertilized and the cells which will become the placenta take over the endocrine secretions, the activity of the corpus luteum gradually wanes, the oestradiol levels fall and eventually the endometrium (lining of the womb) does not get enough hormonal support and is shed in a menstrual bleed. The cycle then starts all over again.

In a pubertal girl, these changes can be followed using ultrasound. In early puberty the signals that are received are not strong enough for single follicles to become dominant. Thus, in a typical cycle, which may last some weeks in, say, a nine year old girl, a crop of follicles is recruited; they all get bigger but none becomes dominant. They all secrete oestradiol and the endometrium increases in size and then as the follicles secrete an amount of oestradiol which is at that time appropriate to suppress FSH everything subsides. These cycles of follicular development occur long before the first signs of puberty and it is only when oestradiol levels are sufficient to promote breast development that we can actually observe that they are happening.

As puberty advances, the swings of oestradiol secretion get bigger, presumably in response to a larger FSH signal generated by a bigger pulse of gonadotrophin releasing hormone. When the oestradiol level is sufficient to produce a substantial amount of endometrial thickening, the endometrium becomes unstable when the level of oestradiol falls and an oestrogen withdrawal bleed takes place. The first of such bleeds is called menarche. It does not infer that ovulation has taken place. Usually it has not, although occasionally it can. Menarche is simply an event which is inevitable if the levels of oestradiol get high enough. This is why in medical terms menarche is not very important because it is an inevitable consequence of ovarian follicular development which is bound to happen one day if the rest of pubertal changes occur normally. In social terms it has assumed a quite disproprotionate importance.

Those with a mathematical mind will have realized that if 20 follicles are recruited every month, something in the order of 250 ova are used up every year in menstrual cycles. If we assume that this happens from the age of ten to the age of fifty when the meopause occurs, it will be seen that a maximum of 10,000 ova are needed for a woman's entire reproductive life. This means that there are 1,990,000 ova unaccounted for from the 2 million that were present at birth. The reason for these sums is shown in Figure 3.3: there is in all women a progessive loss of ova with age and most of the ova with which a woman is originally equipped are never actually recruited but simply atrophy and disappear.

The mechanism by which the follicles themselves govern the menstrual cycle is an immensely ingenious way of ensuring that only one follicle ovulates every month; twins which arise from two ova shed in the same month (unlike twins) are thus relatively rare. It is worth pointing out here that identical twins arise in a quite different way, through a biological accident: at an early stage of cell division the embryo breaks in half into two identical bits and grows into two entire individuals. This accident has nothing to do with reproductive function and occurs randomly, whereas the condition in which two eggs are shed in a single menstrual cycle may happen more than once in a single woman's life and is a familial trait.

Male Reproductive Function

By comparison the acquisition of reproductive function in the male is rather dull. Gonadotrophin releasing hormone pulsation induces gonadotrophin pulsatility which leads to spermatogenesis and testosterone secretion. The former is contingent on the latter in the sense that spermatogenesis can only take place in a seminiferous tubule that is bathed in the testosterone being produced by the surrounding leydig cells. The seminiferous tubules need to be at a slightly

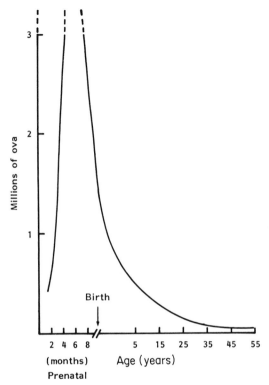

Figure 3.3 The rise and fall of numbers of female germ cells present in the ovaries with age: the shape of this curve is largely independent of reproductive function. The number of ova reaches a peak at about 7 million towards the end of foetal life.

lower temperature than the rest of the body for successful spermatogenesis, which is presumed to be the reason why the testes are located in the scrotum.

There may be cyclical changes in male reproductive function but they are poorly researched and of nothing like so great importance as female cycles. It has, however, been shown that periods of sexual activity bring about their own amplification of the system in that the more sexually active a man may be, the greater will the secretion of the various hormones. The same is not true for women because of the controlling influence of the ovarian follicles.

Growth in Puberty

While the sex steroids, oestradiol from the ovarian follicles and testosterone from the testes, bring about the acquisition of secondary sexual characteristics, the mechanism by which growth occurs in puberty is much more difficult to understand. It may certainly be attributed to the admixture of sex steroid and growth hormone secretion. These clearly interact but each is probably important in its own right. It seems likely that the reason that a girl starts to grow as soon as her breasts start to develop is because LH secretion causes the initiation of steroidogenesis in the ovarian follicle. What this means is that the cells surrounding and lining the follicle are actually secreting androgens, which may be measured in the circulating blood, and these are turned into oestrogens by FSH secretion. In early puberty these androgens would be expected to make a girl grow, to make her skin greasy (which may give her acne), to develop pubic hair and to secrete sweat from under the arms (axilla), which smells different from the sweat of children and is called apocrine, at the same time as the oestradiol levels are rising. Thus, breast development would occur at the same time as androgen mediated growth takes place and the secretion of androgens and oestradiol probably entrains growth hormone secretion.

In the male, the earliest and lowest levels of testosterone are not sufficient to do more than just to make the penis and scrotum grow and some pubic hair appear. The rate of growth in height ceases to decline at this stage of puberty but does not start to increase rapidly until the testes have grown considerably and secrete much more testosterone. At this stage, later in puberty, the boy puts on his adolescent growth spurt and he becomes taller than his female counterpart because of the time which has elapsed between the onset of sex steroid production and the acquisition in his case of levels adequate to increase growth rate.

CONCLUSION

This brief account of the endocrinology of puberty demonstrates how perfectly the human organism is balanced during pubertal development. Each sign of puberty, whether it be breast development, genital development, pubic hair development or the growth spurt, is intimately connected with all the other signs of puberty and it is exceptional for any of them to be out of line. The time over which the changes may take place will be variable, but once the endocrine orchestra is playing, it needs quite a major event to stop reproductive capability from being achieved.

4

The Psychology of Adolescence

The difference between puberty and adolescence has been indicated earlier in this book. Puberty is simply the acquisition of reproductive capability and in primitive societies sexual intercourse began as soon as puberty was considered complete. After a variable period of anovulatory infertility, children were born and the rights and duties of parents were conferred on the individual. Adolescence, therefore, the process of maturing, was not very different in time from puberty. In developed societies, the period between puberty and independence has been increasingly stretched. The minimum school leaving age in the United Kingdom is, for example, at least three years after 50 per cent of girls have started menstruating; the higher the socioeconomic environment of the family, the later the child leaves home and, even when he or she does so, it is probably for a period of further education during which dependence upon the parents is still highly relevant. We have thus extended adolescence to a period of many years during which the conflict between dependence and independence, which is the basis of the psychology of adolescence, persists.

During this period the individual has a number of goals to achieve and it is far from clear how they are best achieved. The complexity of the interdependent variables makes the scientific assessment of this part of growing up extremely complex.

THE GOALS OF ADOLESCENCE

First, and most importantly, the individual has to achieve emotional separation from his family and has to accept responsibility for his or her own affairs in the future. In achieving this 'ego identity' there are continual reminders of the constraints which conflict with this goal of separation. For example, in our society, the constraints of higher education are an obvious barrier to independence and the continuing financial involvement of parents in their children's well-being while this education is taking place merely compounds the problem. Unemployment likewise leads to a continued dependence on parental support.

Secondly, the adolescent has to face the development of appropriate sexuality and the establishment of a personal moral code. In the permissive society in which we live this has probably become more difficult because of the continuous influence of the media in encouraging experimentation with the physical aspects of sexuality without much thought for the emotional commitment. Since initial physical experimentation may not be very successful, and certainly may not be pleasurable for many adolescents, the experience may be extremely disturbing when the expectation of the well-publicized delights of sexual activity is not immediately realized. Making love is not simply a mechanical process.

Thirdly, the adolescent has to develop the ability to relate in an adult fashion to persons outside his immediate family. This is a time for appraisal and it may come as both surprise and a shock to find that an adult individual has no right to love and affection in a way that a child has a right to demand this of its parents. In this respect, leaving home can be a difficult experience because whatever happens to a child in the outside world of school, he or she ought to be able to rely on parents and home to provide a regular emotional recharging of the batteries. When the intervals between recharging become greater, a considerable amount of anxiety may be generated. A child leaving home for the first time may feel very isolated and the conflict between wishing to establish an independent existence and yet needing love and support lands many adolescents away from home for the first time in a very vulnerable situation.

This may be accentuated by finding that those in whom trust has previously been invested by virtue of their family relationship (parents) or public status (such as schoolmasters or doctors) are not always right and they may well fail to measure up to critical inspection when the relationship changes from one of paternalism to an adult relationship between equals. Realization of the necessity to deal with the need for a future vocation and a commitment to attain it brings the adolescent back into the conflicted situation of dependence and independence. The extent to which parents may be involved in career choices and the future of their adolescent offspring may be very difficult in the light of their new adult relationship.

FRIENDS

The choosing of friends in adolescence is of especial importance since they are the basis of separation from the family. Just as the appearance of physical changes of puberty varies enormously in time, so does variation in dating the opposite sex. Parental attitudes are probably not very relevant in this respect but they are important both negatively and positively for the establishment of a peer group. Some adolescents need the approval of parents for the group they choose, while others seek the direct opposite. Parenting obviously becomes very difficult when adolescents experiment with different roles, especially if they consort with groups which seek to develop an identity which is very different from the conventional attitudes of the parents. It seems likely that many who experiment with drugs or gambling or other such activities are really seeking to demonstrate a different identity in the same way that small children may become extremely aggressive in order to demonstrate that they exist.

Parents may make these situations very difficult for their adolescent children. This sometimes occurs because of the way in which all parents relive their childhood through the experience of their own children. It is well recognized that parents treat their children very similarly to how they themselves were treated (battered children become battering parents), and this may lead them to seek vicarious excitement from their children's exploits. Thus while they may on the one hand overtly discourage their children from experimentation with deviant behaviour, they may also, on the other, covertly encourage such activities. One can often sense a frisson of excitement in parents at the exploits of deviant adolescents and such conflicted parenting certainly makes for general unhappiness all round. It certainly leads unscrupulous middle men to offer opportunities for adolescents in terms of drugs and sex which may exploit the division between children and their parents.

SEX

Most adolescents, despite appearances to the contrary, are very ignorant about sexual matters other than the mechanics of sexual intercourse. Most of them, perhaps boys rather than girls, are reluctant to admit this. Most education in sexual matters, apart from learning the parts of the body, is achieved by hearsay from friends and the accuracy of this source of information must often be highly suspect. Thus, much of what an adolescent learns about sex is untrue or at least a mixture of truth and fantasy, and this confusion may even extend to the medical profession.

It is surprising how often otherwise well-qualified doctors lack what seems to be extremely elementary biological knowledge about physical development. For example, many doctors will suggest that intermittent abdominal pain is associated with a developing menstrual cycle long before breast development has occurred, which is clearly a physiological impossibility though not a psychological improbability. The assumption of truth and fantasy in matters sexual is compounded by the fact that reproductive capability long precedes the emotional adaptation which is required for the establishment of a satisfactory relationship.

Such a relationship goes much further than the simple mechanics of sex and demands a degree of commitment for which many adolescents are either unprepared or not prepared to undertake. In this respect, it is my view that the experimentation which is involved in living together without marriage may actually make life difficult. Although marriage entails a legal commitment which may be regarded as a nuisance, it removes a very considerable psychological strain which a common law relationship may entrain. If a couple is simply living together without long-term commitment, there is nothing to stop them from breaking apart, and the least challenge or uncertainty that they are not ideally suited may make them do just this. A successful marital relationship requires constant maintainance and such a relationship is much more able to sustain the ups and downs of everyday life. In other words, the degree of permanence that a legal contract enforces removes a very considerable amount of psychological doubt. It may well be for this reason that preparing for marriage and for having children by living together has not resulted in a fall of the divorce rate: the impermanence of the former relationship may carry through to a lack of commitment in marriage.

The difficulty of establishing satisfactory sexual relationships is considerably increased if there has been disappointment in the first contact and there may then be considerable anxiety in establishing any further relationship. Again parental and peer group pressures may play a part here, either positively or negatively. The process of appraisal with peers may also be extended to a sexual appraisal of the parents. It may be a matter of considerable concern to an adolescent to discover that what had been taken for granted in terms of his parents' relationship may be far from reality. They may have sexual proclivities, both homosexual and heterosexual, which are very surprising to their children. The sexuality of parents is generally distasteful to adolescent offspring and when parents fail to live up to expectations, either in their way of life or their sexual habits, it may be very distressing for all concerned.

WORK

Achievement of independent work status seems to some to be indefinitely prolonged and hedged with so many conditions that its ultimate achievement becomes doubted. The commitment to vocational training of large numbers of adolescents is rather remarkable when one considers its cost in emotional terms. It is of little surprise that pressures are insupportable for some adolescents who then break down and are unable to cope. The pressures to achieve independent work status may, of course, be compounded by parental attitudes, and excessive parental pressure, justifiable or otherwise, may be more than counterproductive. Nevertheless, there are studies which indicate that parental attitudes are still the single strongest factor in governing the ultimate employment of adolescents.

Relatively little research has been done on the part played by 'Saturday jobs' in achieving independence. Certainly the financial independence which such work may provide may be helpful, but many adults forget that the working day of most school children, particularly educationally ambitious ones, may well exceed any working day which would be approved by a government or a trade union. Saturday work adds yet another physical pressure which must be balanced against the other advantages. Such an alternative employment can be psychologically advantageous in providing a relaxation from education, but can also be extremely distracting in terms of mixing with people whose goals and aspirations may be different from those of the Saturday worker.

PARENTAL ATTITUDES

While the goals of adolescence outlined above are difficult for the child to achieve, with or without parental support, parenting is also not easy. Few parents receive any instruction in child rearing and the strongest influence on parenting comes from personal experience. It is a remarkable fact that one has to take a test to drive a motor car or pass an examination to be a doctor but anyone is able in our society to have a child without any qualification at all.

The physical burden of parenting receives little attention but the fact is that a woman of thirty-five having a first child is much less able to stand the sleep deprivation which parenting involves than is her counterpart, say, ten years younger. The same thing necessarily applies to older parents of adolescent children. They are even further away from their own adolescence and may be even less sympathetic to the difficulties which the adolescent finds in establishing his or her identity.

While all parenting is necessarily experimental, the parenting of adolescents must generally be recognized to be a situation which is difficult to win. The compliant adolescent may well never be able to establish a true self-identity and may not be able to establish an adult relationship with his or her parent. In this respect, an adult relationship may be easier to establish with a rebellious adolescent but it seems sad if a physical break in the relationship has to take place before parental nurturing gives way to an adult friendship between parents and children. It is my belief that the fault is more often on the side of the parents.

Some rebuttal of parental attitude is a prerequisite to emotional separation from the family. Nevertheless, such conflict may be highly uncomfortable to an adolescent and a cause of great anxiety which may be greatly magnified in a single-parent situation. In such a situation the demands on the adolescent for emotional support of the parent may actually prevent a normal adult relationship being possible; this may be especially difficult if the adolescent and the parent are of different sex, because there is necessarily a sexual interplay in their relationship. Whether it is better to provide a family home in adolescence, even an unhappy one, or to accept marital separation when 'the children are able to take care of themselves' is outside the scope of this book, but it is an aspect which families in conflict may well need to rehearse.

Finally, there is often a considerable amount of reverse parental pressure on their offspring as the parents get older and more isolated. This, too, may make a satisfactory parent–offspring relationship difficult to maintain in the adult life of the latter. As the extended family becomes reduced in size, whether by death or by separation, the importance of the parent–offspring relationship may become of greater value to the parents than to the offspring. Thus at a time when the adolescent is beginning to establish his or her own identity, parents can be very demanding in terms of requiring friendship to deal with their own advancing age, and they will need to remember that adolescents, like trees in a forest, need to have air to breathe. In proper forest husbandry, the trees are thinned to enable mature specimens to develop. If the parental brambles entwine the developing adolescent, he or she may never be adequately able to separate. This is not a new problem: many of the sons and daughters who have so dutifully looked after their ageing parents were in exactly this situation, and some of them may never have been able to establish a separate and satisfactory independent life in which the goals of adolescence have been achieved. In short, some people never grow up.

ADOLESCENT ATTITUDES

These conflicts, and the realization that there are no winning sides in an adolescent dispute any more than there are in an industrial dispute, take their toll on the adolescent. Both physically and emotionally much is demanded and relatively little is supplied. The adolescent is expected to develop independence in all senses without the means to do so in most. This may not be directly the fault of the parent who may have neither the knowledge nor the means to provide for these needs, but there is little point in complaining about the end result when the preparation for it is inadequate.

Health and education professionals may become involved at all stages in this process, both in normal and deviant behaviour. Their problem is often that their own ability and experience to deal with the situation is lacking because adolescent development is not part of the curriculum of most training courses, medical or otherwise. Further, when adolescent topics are raised in such an environment, many of the teachers and the students find their own personal experience too great adequately to take an objective position. In such situations the attitude of the adolescent may range from the blasé to the truculent and of the professional from aggression to sympathy, but neither is fully understanding of the difficulties that both parents and adolescents experience.

5

Sleep and Energy Requirements

Growth requires a complex interaction between external energy requirements in the form of food and the internal metabolic regulation which is what endocrinology is all about. Both of these factors can be greatly influenced by the emotional climates in which the adolescent finds himself. Food is important in both quality and quantity, particularly at times of rapid growth, and adolescence is certainly one of these. It also, however, has an important cultural aspect which must not be ignored. Few things irritate parents more than when their children do not eat what they wish them to eat, and even toddlers learn that this is the best way to get back at their parents!

There are few data on the relevance of sleep in childhood and such data are urgently needed when one realizes that the primary stimulus to growth hormone secretion is deep sleep and that the gonadotrophin secretion which is crucial for pubertal development occurs mainly at night. What is certainly true is that unhappy children or children with various diseases are known to sleep very badly and this may well influence the rest of their development and they may not grow adequately. Whether this is because they sleep badly or not, we do not yet know.

ENERGY REQUIREMENTS

It is a readily observable fact that different people eat different amounts and this applies equally to children. Many parents have difficulty in adjusting to the fact that the energy requirements of their children may be different from their own. Indeed, so strong is the tendency to impose eating patterns on children that patterns of body fatness are observed to run in families. For a considerable amount of time it was suggested that patterns of body fat were genetically determined, but more careful research has shown that this is almost certainly not the case and that body fat is largely environmentally determined. Within-family resemblances of body shape are due to the sharing of a common environment rather than to a direct genetic influence.

When it comes to feeding children, especially when they reach the adolescent age and begin to establish their own eating patterns, the acceptance of what may be appropriate for them by other adults may set up very serious anxieties. Children learn from the earliest age that food refusal or abnormal eating patterns cause their parents, particularly their mother, great anxiety. One of the commonest reasons why it is difficult to treat obesity in childhood is that mothers simply cannot bear to reduce the calorie intake of their children sufficiently to be effective in terms of weight reduction. While it is relatively easy to recognize this phenomenon between parents and children, especially in other families, it can be very difficult to overcome the problem.

The fact nevertheless remains that food intakes have to be very bizarre in terms of quantity or quality before they have a harmful effect on health. Considering how little control most of us impose on our energy intake, our physical appearance and wellbeing change remarkably little. On the other hand, when eating habits do become so bizarre as to impair health, either in terms of overeating or undereating, help should be sought without delay because the situation is probably already considerably more serious than may be generally appreciated.

There are many widely held beliefs about foods, their

nutritional value and their side-effects. Most of them are incorrect. There is no evidence that eating a high fat diet causes acne or that chocolate causes headaches in the majority of people. There may well be an allergic component to migraine in susceptible subjects but this is not the rule. It is widely believed that carbohydrate foods (bread, potatoes, starch, etc.) are especially fattening: again, this is not true, since it is the fat content of the diet rather than the carbohydrate content that contains the most calories. Finally, there is a widely held view that a large protein intake is 'good for you'. In a Western society, our protein is sufficient many times over, as is also our vitamin intake. Broadly speaking, therefore, adolescents should be allowed to determine their own energy intake and in the majority of instances they will be found to consume a reasonably balanced diet.

SLEEP

The importance of sleep to good health is unquestionable. There are relatively few studies of the sleep pattern of normal adolescents in their home environment. One conducted in my own department by Dr B. J. Taylor indicated a steady decline in total sleep time with age but little difference in terms of deep sleep with age. In other words, the most useful component of our sleep may be a relatively fixed amount and what we enjoy in addition may in some respects be regarded as an added luxury. Dr Taylor's study showed no significant difference between amounts of sleep or sleep stages between males and females and here, as in other aspects, the adolescent is probably best left to get on with whatever he or she prefers. There is little sense in attempting to impose disciplines of sleep on adolescents as long as they are reasonably courteous to other people about them, since this merely sets up antagonism.

EXERCISE

When a subject is as hotly disputed as the importance of exercise, it is likely that there is no clear answer as to what is generally desirable. Some adolescents appear to enjoy and to require intermittent strenuous exercise—others do not. Neither seems to come to any particular harm and there is no hard evidence that either is particularly beneficial to health.

PART II

Normal Adolescence

6

Relationships

Traditionally, the period of adolescence is viewed by adults as one of turmoil and difficulty, and this is largely due to a realignment of previously established relationships. As one adolescent put it to her parents in a family interview with a psychiatrist, 'I'm going through adolescence for the first time and you're going through bringing up an adolescent for the first time.' There are clearly problems on the side of the adolescent and also on the side of the adults with whom he or she may come into contact.

Mention has already been made of the changing role of parents in terms of their adolescent children. It is apparent that some parents and some adolescents find it easier to establish an adult relationship than others, but for those in whom the process is difficult, if not impossible, great sympathy is needed. While divorce of married people is well recognized, separation of parents and children is a more challenging and wounding process. Kindness needs to be the watchword.

RELATIONSHIP WITH PROFESSIONALS

Many adolescents deny that they have 'problems', especially when talking to professionals. Most complain that they are misunderstood and, from their point of view, this may well be true since many of the problems of adolescents are actually the problems of the adults who are having to deal with them. These problems of adults, be they teachers, doctors, social workers or even parents, are particularly confusing for adolescents who are generally educated to believe that most people are working for the common good. The realization that quite a lot are not may come as an unpleasant surprise. Confrontational attitudes by adults may certainly make matters worse. Adolescents need courtesy but an open-ended question may actually be very difficult to handle. In a very simple way, it is less threatening to say to someone 'please sit down' rather than to ask 'do you want to sit down?'. The former is courteous but reassuringly positive. The latter may be polite but it invites many rather different types of reply.

Since all individuals have to come to terms with what may or may not be possible for them to achieve, it is no good for adults to try to solve the unsolvable for an adolescent rather than offering to share the problem. Nor is it any good for parents or other adults to take sides in adolescent conflict. These may be at a purely local (family) level, at school or in terms of politics and the law. It is certainly quite unjustifiable for adults to exploit adolescents in pursuit of their own personal crusades. Attention has already been drawn to parents who get the vicarious excitement from their children's exploits: the same can also be true of other adults, professional or otherwise. On the other hand, it is equally unhelpful of adults, particularly professionals, to wash their hands of the problems of adolescents on the grounds that 'they must make their own decision'. In civilized relationships, there has to be give and take, and this applies especially during the adolescent period.

In short, it seems to be reasonably agreed that adolescents require a positive approach which uses sympathetic but firm authority. In one important study of fourteen year olds in the Isle of Wight, alienation from parents was not found to be common, contrary to popular belief. On the other hand, petty disagreements about clothes, hair and going out were frequently mentioned. Marital disharmony played a significant part in the generation of new disorders appearing in children. There seems to be a growing realization that adolescents are far more positive in their attitude to their responsibilities than they are generally given credit for.

SPECIFIC SITUATIONS

Death

The commonest cause of death in the adolescent age group is traumatic. There is a good reason why insurance companies specify the age of twenty five as being when they cease to apply punitive premiums on motor insurance. The feeling of immortality in adolescence must be recognized, however, as part of the natural exuberance in life, and since we are all more or less continuously at risk from sudden death, overprotection by parents of their adolescent children is likely to be counterproductive.

Nevertheless, adolescents do die of other disorders and various forms of cancer are the commonest cause of such death. Sharing the truth with an adolescent patient is often the best way of dealing with the problem, but many difficulties are actually created by the close relatives of an adolescent when they find it difficult to face the reality of a situation with which the patient has already come to terms. In my experience, many adolescents find the reassurance and security of a hospital ward preferable to being at home during a terminal illness, not so much because they fear their own pain and distress at home but because their problems are taken relatively as a matter of course in hospital while their relationship with their parents and friends at home may be a more or less continuous strain.

Death also occurs in persons surrounding the adolescent: in this case children and adolescents need just as much to go through the reactions of grief as do older persons. Funerals, for example, have an important psychological part to play in the grieving process and it is my belief that children and adolescents suffer much more if they are excluded from the funerals of their relatives in the mistaken idea that they may be upset by them. Being upset is important and protecting a child from upset is often counterproductive. Further, a child excluded from the communal act of grief in which adults have taken part may induce all sorts of fantasy about what has gone on which may take much time to unravel.

Psychiatric Illness

Psychiatric illnesses of adolescents themselves will be considered in Part III but it is important that adolescents are included in discussions about the psychiatric illnesses of those around them. Most adults appear to find it extremely difficult to cope with psychiatric illness in their family: on the whole adolescents seem to understand the problem rather better and they certainly should not be excluded from consideration. In particular, special attention should be paid to the healthy adolescent siblings and children of either physically or psychiatrically ill patients. Many families appear to fall apart after death or illness of a loved one because so much attention has been paid to the sick person that the rest of the family has forgotten to recreate their own relationships. It is all too easy to forget that other people also have feelings and adolescents may be particularly prone to this. Their own problems may be so consuming that they forget that teachers, parents and other professionals need as much emotional support as they.

7

Sexual Function

The physical maturation of the body leads naturally in time to sexual experimentation. It must not be forgotten, however, that the preparedness of the body for such experimentation may be widely distanced in time from the appropriate stage of emotional development. In short, early maturing children may have a considerable problem either in controlling or resisting sexual urges or advances from others from the physical point of view but be quite unable to accommodate the emotional consequences if a sexual relationship is begun at too early an age.

There is no doubt that there is a lot of pressure to become sexually active. Even if it is true that 63 per cent of males and 59 per cent of females at the age of nineteen claim to have been sexually active previously, nearly half of all adolescents will not have been. They are just as normal as anyone else and it is my impression that claims of sexual activity are likely to be grossly exaggerated.

I have seen many girls with late onset of puberty who, in their wish to become mature, have, even in collusion with their mother, fantasized the onset of their periods when uterine bleeding was biologically impossible. This has included at least three patients who were actually born without a uterus, although they did not know it, from whom uterine bleeding was, of course, a physical impossibility. There are high prices to pay from early sexual activity so no adolescent should feel under any obligation to undertake sexual experimentation unless he or she wishes it. Nor should parents interfere in the chronology of this biological function either covertly or overtly.

PROBLEMS FOR BOYS

Since the foreskin separates from the head of the penis during the course of the first year of life there should be no problem by the time of puberty. The foreskin should be fully retractile and indeed should be retracted in order to wash adequately. If the foreskin cannot be drawn back over the head of the penis, medical help should certainly be sought.

By the same token, both testes should have descended into the scrotum long before the onset of puberty. If they are retractile in earlier childhood, that is they naturally assume a position rather high in the scrotum or lower part of the groin, they will descend in puberty. It is, however, important that both testes can be manipulated into the scrotum during childhood, not only because that indicates that they are likely to be functional but also because a retained intra-abdominal testis can develop malignant disease (cancer) later in life. One should know where it is and place it in an observable site or else remove it. If there is any doubt about the correct positioning of the testes, medical advice should be sought.

A not uncommon problem which occurs at all ages, but particularly in adolescence, is torsion of the testis. This is when the testis twists on the spermatic cord and cuts off its own blood supply. If the condition is recognized and treated in time, the spermatic cord can be untwisted and no harm results. If the diagnosis is missed and the treatment delayed, the testis may die as a result of the interruption of its blood supply. In that case, the testis has to be removed and in such a situation it is extremely important to fix the other testis so that it cannot swing on its cord, since this may be a bilateral condition. The key to the mangement of torsion of the testes is early surgical exploration, and it is most important that pain or swelling in the testis be reported within hours for medical advice. About half of the adolescents who present with acute torsion give histories of previous episodes of the same symptoms that have resolved spontaneously. Had these previously been discussed, the ultimate problem might have been avoided.

PROBLEMS FOR GIRLS

The commonest problem for adolescent girls is the regulation of their periods. The onset and mechanism of menstruation has already been discussed and it has been indicated that early menstrual cycles are anovulatory in type. They are thus irregular and can, occasionally, be very heavy. Blood loss due to menstruation in puberty is practically never of a severity to cause anaemia, but the emotional distress of heavy periods may quite outclass the actual degree of loss. Since irregular bleeding in early puberty settles down as soon as the cycles become ovulatory, dysfunctional uterine bleeding is a self-limiting condition which should generally be put up with rather than treated.

Obviously this presumes that the girl is otherwise healthy; if she were to have a bleeding disorder or other blood disease, things might be different and it is certainly worth getting reassurance that heavy periods are actually normal since a simple clinical examination (an internal (vaginal or rectal) examination is not necessary) will normally tell a doctor whether or not there is anything to worry about. In such a situation, it would generally be my view that the consultation and examination by the doctor should be strictly between the adolescent girl and her doctor without parental involvement.

Very occasionally, if the periods are very irregular and then suddenly heavy and if this is likely to interfere with the important life events, such as examinations, interviews or other similar occasions, it may sometimes be justifiable to regulate the flow by a short course of hormonal treatment. Effectively, this involves putting the young girl on a combined oral contraceptive medication which will only rarely be justifiable for this indication. There is hardly ever a place for a gynaecologist to perform a curettage in such a situation, which he might undertake when anovulatory cycles and dysfunctional uterine bleeding occur around the menopause.

D & C is such a commonly performed gynaecological operation that it is worth describing what it actually means. In a D & C, almost always under a general anaesthetic, an instrument is introduced to look up the vagina (a speculum) in order to locate the cervix (neck of the womb). In a nulliparous woman (one who has not had a baby) the cervix is tightly shut and if access to the cavity of the uterus is required, it has to be dilated by a series of blunt ended probes of gradually increasing diameter. This is the dilatation (D) which precedes the scraping out of the lining of the womb (endometrium) leaving the muscular wall of the womb (myometrium) intact. The latter process is called curettage (C). In this way, the contents of the womb are removed very speedily. This is the sort of operation which is performed for an abortion, in which case what is removed from the uterus includes the products of conception. Sometimes, early in a pregnancy, the contents of the womb may be removed in a blind fashion by vacuum extraction, literally sucking out the contents of the womb, in which case the dilation of the cervix does not have to be as great as to allow the introduction of the instrument which is actually used for curettage.

Dysmenorrhea (Period Pain)

It is impossible to assess pain and discomfort experienced by another person, and the distress which the same pain may cause may well be different in different people and may well be affected in the same individual by circumstances emotional and other which have nothing to do with the pain. The onset of menstruation is invested by society with a quite disproportionate importance. Everybody knows that women may have problems around the time of their periods, to such an extent that premenstrual tension has even been used as a defence in court against criminal prosecution. No one who has ever had a tension headache could deny that it is perfectly possible to have physical discomfort without acute organic disease and it is certain that many of the problems which go with menstruation have an important psychological component. This does not mean that the problems do not exist, only that their causation may not be a direct effect of a physical condition.

It is generally believed that anovulatory cycles do not cause dysmenorrhea and most authors report that although the first period may be accompanied by discomfort (for many obvious reasons), subsequent early periods are pain-free. As anovulatory cycles become replaced by ovulatory ones, symptoms of dysmenorrhea may occur. They consist of a cramping lower abdominal pain sometimes associated with nausea, vomiting or diarrhoea, pain in the lower back or thighs or headache.

Measurement of intrauterine pressure in patients with dysmenorrhea shows that there may be muscular spasm in the uterus for reasons which are not clear. The contractions may have to do with chemicals called prostaglandins which are found in the uterus, and it is useful that that universal remedy, soluble aspirin, is not only anti-inflammatory and analgesic (pain relieving), which is why it is superior for toothache to other analgesics which act centrally, but also that it inhibits prostaglandin synthesis. Aspirin is therefore the first remedy for period pains. Most adolescent girls with an explanation of the mechanism and some aspirin will not find their periods too difficult to cope with: others may need more help and the remedy is to block ovulation. This effectively means taking the oral contraceptive pill. This should rarely be necessary.

Dealing with Menstrual Loss

The manufacturers of sanitary towels have, because of the huge market that is involved, not been slow to take advantage of newer materials to construct lighter, smaller and more absorbent products. These will necessarily be what most girls will use. In very early adolescence, there may be considerable difficulty in inserting tampons into the vagina, although the design of these too has considerably improved. Many adolescents will wish to use tampons in order to have as little inconvenience as possible, but it is important to point out that it is dangerous to leave tampons inside the vagina for a long period of time because of the toxic shock syndrome. This condition, which has mainly been seen in the United States of America, is believed to be due to the use of superabsorbent tampons which are left in place for a considerable length of time. Bacteria proliferate in the medium of the tampon and release a toxin which makes the patient extremely ill—indeed some deaths have been reported. Tampons should not be allowed to remain in place for more than about 8 hours, which means that a sanitary towel should generally be used at night.

Amenorrhea

The failure of periods to commence is closely associated with general failure in puberty, and this will be considered in Part III under medical problems. The condition under which periods begin normally and then cease is called secondary amenorrhea, and most of the causes are similar to those outlined in Part III. On the other hand, they should not be overinterpreted. Most girls whose periods are irregular, even if they are very irregular, are perfectly normal, and in an otherwise physically and emotionally healthy adolescent, who is not worried by the lack of periods, more harm is probably done by investigating secondary amenorrhea than waiting for it to right itself by the passage of time, which is much the most likely outcome. There is certainly no justification for regulating secondary amenorrhea by the prescription of hormonal preparations. There has been a widely held view that the administration of hormonal preparations may lead to secondary amenorrhea: in fact, it is much more likely that what has been called post-pill amenorrhea is actually an abnormality of the menstrual cycle which antedated the prescription of the pill and which was regulated by it.

CONTRACEPTION

No topic appears to engender more discussion that this and it is not the purpose of this book to make a moral judgement, rather to make an appraisal of the current scientific situation. Most authorities agree that adolescent pregnancy is not generally a happy state of affairs for the mother and it must be clearly stated that the baby is at considerable risk as well. I doubt whether most sensible people believe that it is wise for an unplanned, unwanted baby to be brought into our already overpopulated world and for the adolescent there are therefore only two choices, not to indulge in sexual intercourse or to use some form of contraception. There can be no middle way. It is certainly most unwise to rely on any form of biological infertility (rhythm methods or the presumption of anovulatory cycles) if sexual intercourse is going to take place. The situation where the tail wags the dog must, however, equally be avoided: just because somebody may have the means of contraception at hand, they must not feel coerced into sexual activity which they may not enjoy, especially as there are considerable dangers of promiscuous sexual activity both immediate and late (see Part III).

There are a number of contraceptive techniques which are available to adolescents without reference to a physician. The first is the condom (a rubber sheath which fits over the penis, often called a french letter) which is one of the oldest methods of contraception used. It has the advantage of providing some protection against sexually transmitted disease and a major advantage of being available for use without preparation. The two main disadvantages are firstly that boys do not like wearing them and secondly that they may be unreliable without an additional spermicidal cream or gel. They may split or come off during the process of sexual intercourse and mechanical failure, although rare, certainly results in quite a lot of pregnancies if couples use this method alone. On the other hand, a condom is greatly preferable to no contraception.

There are various spermicidal vaginal foams, creams and gels but they cannot be relied upon without some other barrier between the sperm and ovum. Such mechanical barriers include the condom for the male and the vaginal diaphragm or cervical (Dutch) cap for the female. These have to be inserted by the girl prior to intercourse and left in place afterwards. The problem with the vaginal diaphragm is that it has to be of the right size for the individual, so a prescription is needed from a Family Planning Clinic. Clearly it has to be inserted before intercourse and some couples find that this removes the spontaneity of sexual activity: even if the woman does not find the insertion of a diaphragm a problem, there are some men who cannot maintain their state of sexual arousal if it is interrupted by the necessity for the girl to insert a diaphragm.

For these reasons, few adolescents and young adults indulging in regular sexual activity choose barrier methods for contraception, but it has clearly to be stated that barrier methods used in association with spermicidal preparations are not only the oldest and amongst the most reliable methods of contraception, but without any question at all by far the safest methods of contraception. The element of safety must not be overlooked in this context.

The intrauterine device (IUD) and the oral contraceptive pill offer additional choices to an adolescent who does not wish to become pregnant. While in theory the IUD is a good choice of contraception for an adolescent, in practice it cannot be recommended to a nulliparous woman. An IUD works by preventing the implantation of a fertilized ovum. In order to do this it has to be placed within the uterine cavity and there is a considerable risk that it will be expelled without the knowledge of the girl. If it is not expelled, it may make menstrual periods heavier and uncomfortable but, most importantly of all, it constitutes a foreign body which may generate infection. The younger the patient, the more likely is infection to be seen with an intrauterine device, and if the infection started by an IUD spreads into the fallopian tubes, inflammation and scarring may result which may cause permanent sterility. For these reasons, the IUD cannot be recommended for the nulliparous woman, particularly as the failure rate is unacceptably high for adolescents. This may be a useful form of contraception for a woman who has a had a baby, who does not wish to have the oral contraceptive pill and cannot make barrier methods work, but who does not mind very much if she were to become pregnant.

This leaves the oral contraceptive pill which, with all its disadvantages, is probably the method which most young people will choose if they mean to have regular sexual intercourse. It is effective and there is minimal risk from pelvic infection as a result of the treatment, although the sexual freedom which the pill confers may be a liability. The long-term worry about prescribing the pill is the risk of cancer. It is probable that the pill can influence cancer in both directions. Carcinoma of the ovary and breast are probably less common in pill users but carcinoma of the cervix and malignant melanoma may be increased by the use of the pill. Carcinoma of the cervix is virtually unknown in those who have never had sexual intercourse and the age at which sexual intercourse begins and the number of sexual partners have a significant influence on the later incidence of carcinoma of the cervix.

The oral contraceptive pill has its effect by replacing ovarian function. Thus, when a patient is taking the oral contraceptive pill, she does not have normal cycles of ovarian follicular development and the normal secretions of her pituitary gland are suppressed. Thus, the pattern of hormonal change which occurs during the course of each menstrual cycle is overridden. When the oral contraceptive pill is started on day 1 of the cycle, a level of oestrogen in the blood is achieved which is somewhere within the range of the early part of the cycle and it is maintained constantly for the succeeding days in which the pill is taken. The endometrium proliferates under the influence of oestrogen, although probably not as much as during a normal menstrual period, and when the oestrogen is removed at the end of the cycle, the endometrium becomes unstable and a brief period of bleeding ensues which either stops spontaneously or is interrupted by the start of another cycle of taking the pill.

For these reasons, periods are regular and pain-free in patients who are taking the pill, but there may be other problems in suddenly imposing an unphysiological level of oestrogen in the blood on a women early in her cycle. The commonest side-effect of taking the pill is water retention, which is manifested by an increase in weight, an increase in girth, a feeling of tightness, headaches and, most seriously, an increase in blood pressure. These symptoms are sometimes sufficient to persuade people to stop the pill, but by judicious alterations of the various constituents within an oral contraceptive pill the side-effects can be minimized. Obviously, millions and millions of women have taken the pill without any serious side-effects for a very considerable period of their lives, and this must be the main justification for advising this as the method of choice for a sexually active adolescent who does not wish to use a barrier method. Nevertheless, the long-term safety of the barrier method does make a lot of sense.

Finally, there is the question of what to do after the event. For an adolescent who presents for care immediately after unprotected sexual intercourse, it is possible to provide a hormonal method of preventing implantation of a possibly fertilized ovum and any family planning clinic will advise. If there is any delay in presentation, this is not possible and the only remedy has to be abortion. Although abortion is thoroughly unattractive in every sense of that word for the patient and the doctor, not to mention the putative father and the surrounding family, it must often be the case that it is preferable to having an unwanted pregnancy. It has clearly to be stated here that there is no alternative to a properly planned (usually minor) surgical procedure early in pregnancy: there may not be a need for a general anaesthetic for an abortion if this is done early, but later on in a pregnancy, a D & C has to be carried out (see above). The earlier in a pregnancy that an abortion is carried out the less traumatic it is, but there is no safe alternative way to interrupting a pregnancy. No girl should try to 'get rid of' a baby without proper medical assistance. To do so is to place the health of the mother in serious risk and if the various methods tried fail, the damage to the baby can be enormous.

8

Behaviour and Personal Habits

It has already been indicated in Part I that the development of independent adult status may place considerable stress on a family. The reasons for this are not hard to understand and much of what is regarded as deviant in adolescent behaviour may be explicable in terms of establishing an independent identity. The attitude of parents towards such behaviour has also been touched upon. In this chapter I wish very briefly to review some of the more common problems of adolescent behaviour.

EARLY AND LATE MATURING

The wide range of onset of puberty has already been mentioned. Life is difficult enough for those who proceed at an average pace through puberty and adolescence but for those who are either very early or very late there may be other difficulties. Early maturers have three common problems. The first is that they may well have been tall throughout childhood and have been treated consistently as if they were older than they actually are. Some children benefit from this, score more highly in examinations and make rapid school progress: others may find it impossible to accommodate the pace demanded and resort to behaviour which one could expect from a child of a much younger age, presumably in order to demonstrate that they are not really as old as they look. For such patients, puberty may bring growth to an end at an early age and other children who continue growing may overtake them both in height and social maturity. Such a patient may apparently begin to fail in all respects and this can create serious anxieties, although these can usually be resolved by an understanding of what is actually going on.

Secondly, early maturing children may be under pressure because the maturation of their body surpasses their emotional development. This may come to a head when opportunities for sexual activity become available and an emotionally unprepared child (more often girls because they mature earlier anyway) may find herself drawn into a sexual relationship, the emotional content of which she cannot contain. Such a situation often precipitates physical symptoms, presumably partly as an indication of a 'cry for help'.

Finally, the early maturing adolescent may consort with an older peer group who may or may not be accepting entirely of the presence of a younger member of the group. Such a person is at danger of not knowing where he or she belongs, to the group of his age or to the group of his maturity; he may get left out altogether by both groups.

The problems of the late maturing adolescent are not dissimilar. The problems of which group to join are obvious. The isolation which a relatively immature adolescent may endure may be very hard to take and adolescents are by no means forgiving in their attitude to those who do not measure up to peer group standards. This sort of unhappiness can very severely affect progress at school and as it comes at an age (sixteen to eighteen) which is crucial for educational attainment and for future job prospects and careers, the need for prevention of this difficulty is great. Such prevention may be purely physical, that is physical maturity may be advanced by some sort of therapeutic means, or it may be psychological. Prevention of both types may be needed but the important thing is that parents and adolescents in this situation should know that something can be done for them, if they only ask in the appropriate place.

The first person to approach is probably the family doctor, although in most situations where there are large numbers of adolescents (e.g. university halls or colleges) there are often self-referral clinics. If the family doctor will not listen or accept that there is a problem, the parent or adolescent must demand a second (preferably specialist) opinion.

FOOD

There is a growing awareness that food plays an important part in promoting good health. Many adolescents and, regrettably, many parents appear to think that eating for health is something which only applies to the middle aged. Of course, nothing could be further from the truth. Eating a low fat, high fibre diet has been shown to prevent coronary heart disease and stroke in adult patients so it is certainly very much better if such dietary habits begin in childhood. The basis of a healthy diet is shown in Table 8.1 and if adolescents would tend towards this sort of sensible eating, they would do themselves much good in the long run.

ALCOHOL, TOBACCO AND OTHER DRUGS

The psychological pressures to demonstrate adult behaviour through the use of alcohol and tobacco are very strong and there can be few adolescents who will not experiment with both. It is hypocritical and pointless for doctors to pronounce upon these habits but it is worth briefly setting the context in which they may be seen.

The extent to which alcohol impairs performance is greatly underestimated by most adults. A celebrated

Table 8.1 Table of sensible eating

Foods to be encouraged	Foods to be taken in moderation	Food to be discouraged
Unsweetened fruit juices, tea, coffee, water	Milk, custard	Milk drinks, sweet drinks of all types, cream
Puffed wheat, Shredded wheat, Weetabix	Cornflakes, Rice Crispies	Sugar-coated cereals, sweetened muesli
Wholemeal bread, flour, biscuits		White bread, flour, biscuits
Home-made soups		Packet and tinned soups
Fish, poultry, game	Eggs, grilled lean meats	Fried fish and meat, fish fingers, fish cakes
All vegetables including: jacket potatoes, haricot beans, lentils, etc.		Vegetables cooked in fat, potato crisps
Raw whole fruit and jelly made from unsweetened fruit juice	Fresh fruit salad	Tinned or stewed fruit
Cottage cheese	Hard cheeses	Cream cheese and cheese spread
Natural yoghurt		Fruit-flavoured yoghurt
Lemon juice	Vinaigrette dressing	Mayonnaise

experiment on the effect of alcohol in doses way below those required for the legal limit of alcohol permitted for driving, let along intoxication, on the driving skills of Birmingham bus drivers showed clearly that a little alcohol may be seriously deleterious to performance. Most musicians will confirm that this is the case and it is a pity that it is not more widely appreciated that, whatever the feelings to the contrary, performances are rarely improved by alcohol and that the removal of inhibition by mild intoxication is seldom beneficial. The same is not so for an audience, which is why a good (sober) after-dinner speaker is appreciated.

The effects of heavy drinking in terms of cirrhosis of the liver, liver cancer and brain atrophy are well known but the effects of lesser intakes of alcohol on calorie consumption and the genesis of obesity are often overlooked. Middle aged spread is often the consequence of affluence and alcohol and is certainly not a physiological occurrence. On the other hand, lest these comments be taken as advocacy for temperance, it should also be recognized that a small intake of wine (about a glass a day) has been shown to have a positively beneficial effect on health. It should be emphasized that the amount of alcohol an individual can safely consume appears to be closely associated with his muscle mass: since men have more muscle than women, women are particularly at risk from abuse of alcohol. Alcohol should not be consumed by a pregnant woman: the effects of even very small amounts of alcohol on the developing foetus may be very severe.

The well-publicized risks of cigarette smoking for the development of cancer appear to have been widely understood. What has not been appreciated is that the effects of tobacco smoking are far more important in terms of chronic bronchitis and cardiovascular disease (heart attacks and strokes) than they are for cancer. Smoking is also extremely bad for a developing foetus and this is presumed to be due to the direct toxic chemical effects of tobacco as well as a decrease in the oxygen carrying power of the maternal blood. Unfortunately, there is almost nothing that can be said in favour of smoking, which is presumably why the idea that smoking is normal is being discouraged and non-smoking areas are becoming the norm.

It is widely held that the taking of marihuana (cannabis, pot, hash, etc.) is not in fact different or more harmful than either of the two preceding habits. This may well be the case, since marihuana is not a drug of addiction but one of habituation, that is that one does not have to take an increasing amount for the same effect, which is what characterizes an addictive preparation. There are many, including myself, who find it baffling that the legal sanctions on the taking of pot should be so much greater than those on the taking of alcohol or tobacco. The major argument is that the purchase of marihuana brings susceptible individuals into association with the purveyors of the more destructive addictive drugs such as opium, cocaine, heroin, etc. The fact of the matter, of course, is that if marihuana were legalized, there would be no question of coming into contact with drug pushers, any more than buying a packet of cigarettes in a corner shop involves drug trafficking. The medical truth of the matter nevertheless remains that there are no demonstrable benefits from taking marihuana, save for a group identity, and there are probably other and more preferable ways to seek peer group approval than through this particular avenue.

Addiction begins when a child is offered a drug, usually by someone they know, and accepts. For the most part this is a one-off occasion and only a very few will become addicted; for them deep sympathy is needed followed by action.

Nobody knows why most people can take alcohol, tobacco, morphine and many other substances when they wish to do so but do not need to do so when they do not, while just a few individuals are 'hooked'. The dangers (and expense) of becoming hooked on drugs of addiction are so great that a mature individual will see no very good reason for experimenting. One does not need to put a hand into a fire to imagine what getting it burnt is like and the same must necessarily be true of these extremely potent and dangerous substances. There are, of course, actual physical dangers from drugs which are injected and from hallucinatory drugs (LSD, etc.) which further complicate the issue. Anybody who is having problems in this sort of area would be well advised to seek expert help.

PART III

Medical Problems

9

Problems of Entering Puberty

Reference to Figure 3.2 and the accompanying discussion on page 31 will indicate that there has to be normal function of the hypothalamus, the pituitary gland and the testes or ovary for a child to enter puberty normally. There can be disorders of function at any level.

Much the commonest problem is that a person is just late in development. I have already indicated that 97 per cent of girls and boys are showing some signs of puberty by their fourteenth birthday, but this still leaves 3 per cent who have not done so by that time, and it is perfectly possible to show no signs of puberty whatsoever until the age of sixteen and yet to be perfectly normal. On the other hand, it is obvious that the longer the lapse of time becomes, the less likely it is to be normal. This is why it is well worth consulting an expert earlier rather than later. In the majority of cases, some changes are obvious to the expert which form the basis of an authoritative prediction of what is going to happen. Further help can be given if things do not progess as predicted, and it is certainly not good enough for an adolescent with pubertal delay just to be told that all will be well one day.

In growth and development, consonance is the rule. By this I mean that an adolescent who is going late into puberty is likely to have delayed growth as well as delayed puberty. He or she is therefore likely to be small in relation to peers and will almost certainly have delayed skeletal maturation, meaning that there is plenty of time for growth in height to occur when puberty starts. In other words, a child who is tall and showing no signs of puberty is much less likely to be normal than a child whose growth and development is delayed in all respects. The pattern of growth during childhood can be extremely helpful in assessing this sort of problem and in distinguishing it from the other causes of delayed puberty which will be mentioned below. It is a matter of considerable regret that few children have adequate records kept of their growth during childhood

Pathological disorders of puberty (Table 9.1) begin with disorders of the hypothalamus. It has already been indicated that the hypothalamus has to produce gonadotrophin releasing hormone in a pulsatile fashion for puberty to be initiated and reproductive function maintained. Exactly what causes the gradual increase in the hypothalamic signal that brings about sufficient gonadotrophin secretion to induce puberty is not known but any serious and prolonged illness may well cause pubertal delay. Such illnesses can also cause arrest of pubertal development which is, if anything, more serious than pubertal delay, since it excludes those with simply a problem in timing.

The systemic illnesses which are particularly likely to cause pubertal problems are mainly those associated with poor states of nutrition. Anorexia nervosa, which will be discussed on page 116, is very important and may not always be obvious, especially if the child actually eats but then secretly vomits. This condition, called bulaemia, is probably considerably more common than is generally realized. Organic causes of malnutrition are also important, however, and gastrointestinal disease (Crohn's disease, ulcerative colitis, coeliac disease), liver problems, renal disease and respiratory problems (especially undertreated asthma) are all important in this respect. Whether they actually delay puberty through the disease process itself or through undernutrition

Table 9.1 Causes of late puberty

Origin	Late puberty
Hypothalamic	GNRH deficiency, isolated or associated with other deficiencies, with or without a structural abnormality Emotional causes, e.g. anorexia nervosa Systemic illness
Pituitary	Space-occupying lesion, e.g. prolactinoma Post-operative gonadotrophin deficiency Idiopathic with or without hyposmia (e.g. Kallman's syndrome)
Gonadal	Anorchia Gonadal dysgenesis with or without chromosomal abnormality Disorders of sex hormone biosynthesis
Adrenal	Congenital adrenal hyperplasia (cholesterol desmolase deficiency 3β-hydroxysteroid dehydrogenase deficiency, 17α-hydroxylase deficiency) Congenital adrenal hypoplasia (associated with gonadotrophin deficiency)
Idiopathic	Mainly in boys

is not clear, but certainly a sick person does not develop in puberty.

There are two special endocrine disorders which may cause delay in puberty due to a lack of hypothalamic activity. The commonest of these is diabetes mellitus. Diabetes in adolescence will be discussed on page 141 and the psychological problems that cause the delay in puberty is not known, but getting either or both under control certainly causes satisfactory maturation in puberty. Deficiency of thyroid hormone also causes lack of puberty. Sometimes breast development may be seen in girls, but without the accompanying growth spurt and appearance of pubic hair; in boys, there may be some testicular enlargement which is disproportionate to other signs of puberty. These features are characteristic of hypothyroidism but are often not picked up by doctors.

Apart from the nutritional disorders and the problems secondary to other endocrine disease, disorders of the hypothalamus itself are not uncommon. There may be deficiency of either just gonadotrophin releasing hormone or of the other hormones in varying combinations. Usually these deficiencies are idiopathic, the grand name that doctors give to conditions they do not understand. It must be presumed that most hypothalamic releasing hormone deficiencies are due to a congenital absence of the relevant secretory cells.

The secreting cells can, however, be destroyed by other processes. A tumour around the area of the hypothalamus may have very serious endocrine effects, but the commonest cause of organic gonadotrophin releasing hormone deficiency is radiotherapy for other intracranial malignant diseases. If a child has a brain tumour and a large amount of irradiation has to be given to cure the child, one of the consequences of the irradiation may be destruction of endocrine cells in the hypothalamus. This commonly causes growth hormone releasing deficiency.

As well as an actual lack of gonadotrophin releasing hormone there may also be problems in its pulsatile secretion. Unless gonadotrophin releasing hormone is released in gradually increasing amounts at about 90 minute intervals, puberty does not occur satisfactorily. There can be problems either with the timing of the pulses or with their size. Occasionally, the increasing size of the pulse appears to become arrested and puberty then stops at whatever stage it has reached. This seems to be a rather common cause of infertility in both adult men and women. They have achieved some development of secondary sexual characteristics but have not managed to reach full reproductive capability.

From the point of view of doctors, sorting out problems of the secretion of hypothalamic releasing hormones is quite a problem. A doctor can administer the releasing hormone and see whether the pituitary is capable of responding to it, but this does not tell him very much about the pattern of secretion of the releasing hormone. What he has to do is either measure it directly (which is not actually possible at the time of writing) or to measure the pituitary hormone responses during the course of a 12 to 24 hour period. This necessitates very frequent blood sampling and is tedious and time consuming for all concerned. Fortunately, in girls, a short-cut is provided by ultrasound imaging of the ovaries and uterus. This technique requires special skill but the appearances of the pelvic organs tally extremely well with the blood hormone levels to such an extent that the latter can be omitted in the majority of instances. A very specialized medical service is, however, needed for the economical investigation and management of these problems. Most centres have insufficient experience upon which to draw.

PITUITARY DISORDERS

The pituitary gland is the slave of the hypothalamus and unless it is either congenitally absent or destroyed, it is likely to produce gonadotrophins if the hypothalamus is intact. Even if high-resolution radiographic studies fail to demonstrate much pituitary tissue, repeated stimulation by a small amount by gonadotrophin releasing hormone can be sufficient to induce puberty. Pituitary aplasia (complete lack of pituitary gland) should have been detected much earlier in childhood through the secondary effects on growth and well-being.

If the pituitary formed normally during intrauterine life, it can be destroyed later. Sometimes this happens through an event we cannot explain but more commonly destruction is by a tumour or by the surgery that is required to remove the tumour. The consequent lack of gonadotrophins means that puberty cannot be entered normally, but the lack of the other pituitary hormones also requires attention, especially because the interaction between the use of growth hormone on the one hand and the induction of puberty on the other is very relevant to these patients. Wherever possible, patients in such situations should not be made to wait for puberty induction in the mistaken belief that they will do better in the end if they have growth hormone for some time and then have induction of puberty. Growth in adolescence demands the combination of sex steroids and growth hormone and both should be given at once.

GONADAL DISORDERS

The final common pathway by which the hypothalamus and pituitary bring about the actual changes of puberty is through the secretion of gonadal steroids. If the ovaries or testes have not formed properly, there can, of course, be no puberty. A much less common problem is that there is a defect in the synthetic process by which the sex steroids are made. This, too, will affect advance in puberty.

It is unusual for testes which have descended into the scrotum not to function normally. In order to descend

during foetal life and infancy, they have to be able to secrete testosterone in response to hypothalamo-pituitary signals and therefore if they are descended they must have been
capable of secreting testosterone. If they are not descended,
however, there may well be a problem. The failure of one
testis to descend is not so important in this context. This
is usually due to the fact that, as the testis passes from the
abdomen to the scrotum through the inguinal canal in the
groin, it gets off its normal path and may be located in the
groin. An operation called an orchidopexy has then to be
done to place it in the proper position. This should be done
at least before school age and certainly before the age of ten
years so that testicular maturation can take place with the
testis in the scrotum. One testis will, however, be perfectly
sufficient if there is any problem in the actual operation.

Bilateral undescent of the testes (cryptorchidism) is much
more serious. It is very unlikely that the same accident of
descent will have occurred to both testes; if neither has descended, it strongly suggests that there may be a problem
with the hypothalamus, the pituitary or with the testes themselves. It is important here to differentiate between truly
cryptorchid testes, which may be intra-abdominal or may
just have started their descent in the inguinal canal, and
testes which are retractile. The latter are testes which have
descended normally but which rise to the neck of the scrotum and may be difficult to find but which are otherwise
normal and will come down when the appropriate hormonal
signs occur in late prepuberty. The administration of gonadotrophin will mimic this situation and a normal retractile
testis which secretes testosterone will descend.

In true cryptorchidism, the higher the testes are found,
the less likely they are to function normally in puberty.
All boys who have bilateral cryptorchidism (and there are
not very many who genuinely come into this category)

should have detailed endocrine assessment, preferably before surgery, to define the endocrine situation and determine whether there is functioning testicular tissue present. The operation should not simply be done and the boy left possibly to go into puberty or possibly not, depending upon whether or not he is actually normal. Bilateral cryptorchidism is a serious condition which should not just be operated on and forgotten.

Although the presence of a testis in foetal life is necessary for male sexual development, it is possible for testes subsequently to disappear (so-called vanishing testes). This obviously makes normal development in puberty impossible and is part of the differential diagnosis of bilateral cryptorchidism. The operation which may be undertaken to find such testes may be very extensive, which is why a test to detect the presence of functioning testicular tissue is important before such an operation is undertaken. Whether non-functioning testicular tissue should be explored and removed is debated and the opinion of an expert is needed in such a situation.

In girls, the counterpart to absence of the testes is absence of the ovaries. It is rare for the ovaries not to form properly: what usually happens in ovarian (gonadal) dysgenesis is that the ovaries form normally but the usual loss of ovarian germ cells with age (Figure 3.3) is greatly accelerated so that the girl has become menopausal before she reaches puberty. This may occur as an isolated event, when the girl has a normal chromosome constitution, but it may also be associated with chromosomal disorders. In the commonest of these, the Turner syndrome, there is a lack of one female (X) chromosome. As a considerable amount of the genetic material which is concerned with the determination of height is carried on the X chromosome, girls with the Turner syndrome not only lack ovarian function but are also short. They can have other body features which are associated with the condition, but short stature and ovarian failure are much the most important.

In patients with the Turner syndrome who have no treatment, the average final height is 142 cm (4ft 8in) and there is a spread of height around this which is determined by the heights of the parents. Because this condition is quite common, a lot of effort has been expended in trying to get girls with this condition taller. They suffer from growth hormone deficiency more often than most children but it is possible that even those who are not growth hormone deficient will benefit from additional growth hormone. This method of treatment is currently being tried. There are other medications which are available for treatment to increase height: one used widely in all parts of the world is Oxandrolone. The long-term benefits of this medication are hotly disputed but it is my belief that it is effective if it is used in proper combination with oestrogens to induce puberty and generate a maximal pubertal growth spurt. What is certainly important is that the parents of a girl with Tuner syndrome should seek the opinion of a paediatric endocrinologist *early* in the management of their child's condition, well before the normal age of puberty. Few paediatricians or gynaecologists and endocrinologists in adult practice see sufficient numbers of these patients to be fully up to date with all the advances which are occurring. Final height can only be influenced by seeing and treating such patients before the need to induce puberty.

Other chromosomal constitutions can also be seen in girls with gonadal dysgenesis. If the chromosomal constitution is normal female, there is no problem with height, but puberty has to be induced in the manner which will be described below. If, however, there is a Y (male) chromosome present, it may be inferred that it was inactive and failed to cause the development of a testis. The gonad has then remained rudimentary. Since there was no male sex hormone during foetal life, the patient has normal female external genitalia and a uterus but has primitive gonadal streaks where she should have ovaries. There is a danger that such gonadal streaks may turn malignant and they should be removed before the patient enters her teens.

The presence of a Y chromosome in an otherwise normal looking girl may result in another disorder of pubertal development, testicular feminization or androgen insensitivity. In this condition, a testis forms normally and secretes testosterone in foetal life. Because there is an inherited deficiency of testosterone receptors in the relevant tissues, the male external genitalia fail to form. On the other hand, the second hormone which the foetal testis has to secrete, the antimüllerian hormone, functions normally and prevents the development of the uterus, the fallopian tubes and the upper part of the vagina. At puberty, such patients have normally active testes but since the testosterone can have no effect, because of the lack of tissue receptors, it is converted into female sex hormone (oestradiol) and this causes development of quite normal breast tissue. Because there are no testosterone receptors, pubic hair is absent and no menstruation can occur because there is no uterus present.

Such patients thus present as normal looking girls with normal breast tissue but with a short vagina, no pubic hair and a lack of periods. There is a danger in such patients of malignant change in the intra abdominal testes and, in former days, the testes were removed. This is now thought not to be a good idea because they act as a useful source of oestrogen. Through the development of ultrasound imaging, it is possible to locate and to keep an eye on the testes and to leave them in place, thus avoiding the necessity for oestrogen replacement treatment.

Finally much less common than these disorders of gonadal development are the various abnormalities of sex steroid biosynthesis which may occur. Since these may also effect steroid biosynthesis in the adrenal glands, they may become evident before puberty. If they do become evident at puberty, it is because pubertal development does not proceed at all or because it proceeds in an abnormal fashion, for example the development of breasts in an otherwise normal male. Since none of these disorders is very common, they really do deserve the attention of a specialist in this field.

TREATMENT

The diagnosis of disorders of delay in sexual development requires the testing of the hypothalamo-pituitary-gonadal axis and the definition of where the problem has occurred. This requires the skills of a specialist in this area who needs not only access to hormone measurements but also clinical and growth assessment facilities. For the investigation of girls, the use of ultrasound examination to determine the size and appearance of the ovaries and uterus has enormously simplified investigation. The range of facilities required make the whole process much more straightforward in a specialized department: this is not an area for the amateur physician.

Treatment will be dictated by the diagnosis; it is much easier to treat than to diagnose, but treatment should aim to follow a physiological time scale. Thus the induction of puberty ought to take not less than eighteen months and probably rather longer than this. Unless adolescents are going to wait an excessively long time to become sexually mature, treatment must necessarily begin early, certainly not after the fourteenth birthday. If treatment is delayed beyond this age, the danger is that an unphysiological time scale will be adopted, which is bad from every point of view, but especially bad for the cosmetic results, for the growth which can be achieved and for the time available for emotional adaptation to puberty.

There is one (and only one) disadvantage in the employment of treatment early and this is that a patient who might ultimately develop in puberty might be treated unnecessarily. The reason for this is that it is still very difficult to distinguish between a timing problem regarding the onset of puberty and true deficiency of gonadotrophin releasing hormone. This distinction may be able to be made through gonadotrophin profiles but it may well be in the interest of a patient with simple delay of puberty to be treated, even if this is not strictly necessary, because of the distress that the pubertal delay incurs. Such a patient has the additional advantage that when treatment is complete, no maintenance treatment for maintaining sexual function will be needed, whereas patients with gonadotrophin releasing hormone deficiency will not be in such a happy situation. In this situation, there is nothing wrong with treating first and making the diagnosis later.

The most physiological treatment is clearly the administration of gonadotrophin releasing hormone in a pulsatile manner designed to reproduce the course and duration of normal puberty. Using a pump such as that illustrated in Figure 9.1 this is certainly possible. Very small doses of gonadotrophin releasing hormone have to be given by subcutaneous injection at night in the first instance and the dose of gonadotrophin releasing hormone has to be increased first at night and then given during the day as well. While it is obviously inconvenient to have to use a pump, the advantage of this treatment is that it entirely mimics normal puberty. Whether or not this is necessary for fertility in the long term is not yet clear.

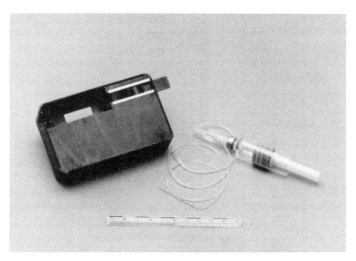

Figure 9.1   A hormone infusion pump. (Courtesy of Dr Ian Sutherland, National Institute of Medical Research)

For patients who have no putuitary gland, it will probably not be possible to use this form of treatment and in these instances it may be necessary to use gonadotrophins themselves. This applies especially to patients who have actually had surgical removal of the pituitary gland because in patients with congenital hypopituitarism, there is probably sufficient pituitary tissue present which can be stimulated to grow by repeated administration of gonadotrophin releasing hormone. Again which treatment is superior in the long term is under active consideration at present.

When gonadotrophins are used, they can generally only be used in boys. The administration of gonadotrophins to girls is too complicated for practical purposes since it leads to excessive follicular growth, ovarian follicular cyst development and the secretion of oestrogens in an erratic fashion which leads inevitably to irregular vaginal bleeding. In boys, preparations which contain LH are given in the first instance to stimulate the production of testosterone and at a later stage preparations containing LH and FSH are added. In this way, spermatogenesis should be achieved. This treatment involves injections at about weekly intervals over a long period of time.

In girls with pituitary or gonadal disorders and in boys with testicular problems, the only treatment which is available for the induction of secondary sexual characteristics is the employment of sex steroids. Technically, this is not the same as inducing puberty, since reproductive capability cannot be achieved. Nevertheless, it has to be the choice of therapy in a substantial number of patients. Since it is the simplest treatment available, it will be important in the future to determine whether such treatment has any consequences for the induction of fertility in the long term. The indications are that it does not have such consequences, which means that there may be no advantages in the more complicated therapeutic regimens for the administration of GnRH or gonadotrophins.

Once again, the principles of mimicking a physiological time scale are needed and *very* small doses of testosterone or oestradiol should be introduced in the first instance and *very* gradually increased in order to mimic the rising levels of sex steroids which occurs in normal individuals as puberty advances. As long as treatment is begun in time and the increase is gradual, the cosmetic end result in terms of secondary sexual development is satisfactory.

EARLY PUBERTY

Although it is the lack of pubertal development which is likely to cause problems in adolescence, it is worth just sparing a thought for those whose sexual development is precocious. The causes of such early development are shown in Table 9.2. Their investigation and management is outside the scope of this book. They are sufficiently unusual to make it important for children with precocious development and to be seen in departments which specialize in the field.

Table 9.2 Causes of early puberty

Early puberty	Origin
Intracranial space-occupying lesion	Hypothalamic
Raised intracranial pressure	
Mental retardation	
McCune–Albright syndrome (probably hypothalamic)	
Hypothyroidism	Pituitary
Ectopic source of gonadotrophin (e.g. Hepatoblastoma in boys)	
Functioning tumours	Gonadal
Drug ingestion	
Congenital adrenal hyperplasia (21-hydroxylase, 11β-hydroxylase deficiencies)	Adrenal
Adrenal neoplasm	
Cushing's syndrome	
Mainly in girls	Idiopathic

Early pubertal development—pubertal development before the age of eight years—has two main disadvantages. The first is that puberty comes at a time when the individual is emotionally unable to cope with the physical changes. In boys libido (sexual drive) may be a considerable problem. In girls, the early onset of menstruation may cause problems at primary school. The second problem concerns that of growth: the average boy gains about 30 cm from the time of the onset of puberty and the average girl about 25 cm. If the child is not adequately tall by the time he or she starts to develop in puberty, final height may be severely compromised.

Treatment is available to deal with the development of the secondary sexual characteristics. This can be either by eliminating gonadotrophin secretion altogether or by abolishing the pulsatility of gonadotrophin secretion. Different agents act in different ways but either way secondary sexual maturation is halted. Unfortunately, no method has yet been found which reliably increases final height, although current information regarding the use of medications directed solely at gonadotrophin secretion looks hopeful.

By the time that these patients enter the adolescent age group, their problems are really at an end, except for their short stature. Once their peers catch them up in terms of sexual maturation there is clearly no need for further treatment.

10

Physical Problems Associated with Puberty

GYNAECOMASTIA

Just as there are changes in the female breast at puberty, changes that are usually welcome, there are also changes in the male breast. This is not at all surprising since there is certainly as much oestrogen available to a boy in early puberty as to a girl. Indeed, it is more of a mystery that there is not much more development of the male breast at puberty than that the female breast develops. It is believed that the reason why the male breast does not develop so much is that there is testosterone (male sex hormone) opposing the action of oestrogen and it is certainly true that in situations where testosterone production is severely deficient, breast development is quite marked. Nevertheless, even in normal boys, there is always some breast enlargement around the time of puberty.

In the vast majority of cases, this disappears spontaneously. It may, of course, appear to be exaggerated in boys who are already obese and anxiety in these boys may be heightened by the fact that there is also a lot of fat over the pubic bones. This fat may conceal the true length of the penis. In such a situation, doctors may also fear that there is a problem in male sexual development because of the apparent small size of the penis and the amount of breast enlargement. In fact, careful examination usually reveals a perfectly normal penis, normal size testes and breasts which are largely fat.

However, even normal breast development sometimes causes embarrassment, and if a boy is well advanced in puberty and yet has large breasts, some thought should certainly be given to them. It is usually possible on simple clinical examination to exclude a disorder where there is inadequate secretion of testosterone, and this can certainly be readily sorted out by some simple blood tests. Where there is no such lack, which is much the most likely, it is generally preferable to resort to surgical removal of the breast tissue, which is done through a very small incision just below the nipple which heals without leaving any signs at all, rather than to leave the boy to suffer from breast enlargement which may be a considerable embarrassment. When such surgery is undertaken, it is worth having an endocrinological assessment at the same time to exclude one of the disorders of sexual development which may be manifested by breast enlargement. A full description of these disorders is outside the scope of this book but may be found in the author's *Clinical Paediatric Endocrinology* (Blackwell Scientific Publications, 1981).

Breast disorders also occur in pubertal girls. The absence of breast tissue requires the full appraisal of disorders of pubertal development (Part III, Chapter 9). Whatever the cause of pubertal failure may be, a girl must be reassured that with the slow introduction of oestrogen therapy, breast development will be normal. It is most important to emphasize the word 'slow'; too many girls are given much too large a dose of oestrogen because they are only treated when they are relatively old and this is undesirable from many points of view, not least the fact that the breasts develop very badly in such a situation. No girl should be given more than 5 μg of ethinyl oestradiol at the start of treatment for delayed breast development.

Asymmetrical breast development is a common occurrence. There is often development of one breast before the other and some minor degrees of inequality in size are really quite common. Serious degrees of inequality are generally transitory and no treatment should be contemplated until the breasts are fully mature. If at this stage there is severe breast inequality, it is necessary to undertake either surgical enlargement of one breast or reduction of the other to make them equal in size.

Rarely, breast asymmetry may result from a complete absence of the breast on one side which may be combined with a lack of the underlying muscle. Surgical correction for this deformity is necessary. Lesser degrees of breast hypoplasia can also be treated with a surgical approach (augmentation mammoplasty) and all girls who are unhappy with their breast development should receive sympathetic consideration for these types of operation, since abnormal breast development may be a serious handicap in establishing a satisfactory sexual relationship with the opposite sex. Girls should, however, be assured that the appearance of the breast normally bears very little relationship to how it will function after a child has been delivered. Some of the smallest breasts actually lactate most effectively.

Finally, there is the question of excessive breast development. To some extent beauty in this respect is in the eye of the beholder but there are certainly some girls in whom very large breasts may develop and these may be not only uncomfortable but also unsightly. Operations to reduce the size of breasts are possible but they are difficult to perform and end up with a normal looking breast which functions normally. In general, therefore, surgeons tend rightly to be very conservative about recommending operations to reduce large breasts unless the problem is extreme. In this respect, it is worth mentioning that a girl who becomes very obese around the age of puberty may develop very large breasts which may be considerably unsightly. Unfortunately, loss of weight later does not enable the breast to regain a normal contour. It is important, therefore, to avoid the rapid onset of obesity around the age of puberty.

Occasionally the breasts secrete a milky discharge, particularly if they are stimulated. This is called galactorrhoea and is most commonly associated with pregnancy, a diagnosis which must be excluded before any other investigations are undertaken. It is certainly worth consulting medical advice about galactorrhoea in an otherwise normal girl.

HAIR DEVELOPMENT

The normal development of pubic hair results in both sexes from the secretion of androgens from the adrenal glands, associated in boys with secretion of testosterone from the testes. As testosterone is a necessary precursor for the synthesis of oestradiol in the ovarian follicle, there is probably a contribution to pubic and axillary hair growth in normal girls from this source. There is no doubt, however, that oestrogens play a facilitative role in the growth of hair. Although most girls with the Turner syndrome (absence of the ovaries) do show a little development of pubic hair before they receive any oestrogen treatment, the introduction of oestrogens to induce breast development produces a sudden increase in the amount of pubic hair.

A total absence of pubic hair in a boy is nearly always associated with one of the disorders of puberty which have been covered in Chapter 9, since it is impossible for a boy to mature in other respects and not to have any pubic hair. The same is not true for girls and the major cause is testicular feminization or androgen insensitivity which has already been described (page 92).

Axillary hair (hair in the armpit) usually grows rather later than pubic hair. Occasionally, particularly in females, axillary hair may be seen before pubic hair. This is usually due to a benign condition of the adrenal glands called premature adrenarche but it is worth making the point that the onset of puberty, particularly in girls, is associated with the secretion of apocrine sweat which is much more offensive than sweat that comes from the sweat glands not in the apocrine areas. This is why body odour occurs in adults and not in children. Many mothers are worried about body odour (with or without hair) in their prepubertal children. They should be encouraged to treat the matter exactly as they do their own body in this respect. Some mothers worry that to shave the axilla or use deodorants will cause problems but in the context of a whole life of use, a year or two is quite unimportant. It is certainly considerably better than allowing the child to be teased at school on this account.

Unwanted hair elsewhere on the body is quite common at puberty. Few boys worry about excessive hair growth on the trunk or face but it can be a source of great unhappiness to girls. Unfortunately it is true to say that doctors are extremely ineffective at treating hirsutism (medical name for excessive hair) and it can become a serious problem. Occasionally, such patients are helped by medication and it is certainly worth consulting an expert before resorting to cosmetic treatment of the beauty parlour type in a young girl.

Hirsutism can develop as an isolated finding but may be associated with other disorders of puberty such as irregular menstrual function or other evidence of male sex hormone secretion such as severe acne, a voice change and so on.

Some increase in facial and body hair nearly always accompanies pubertal development but excessive growth certainly requires careful clinical evaluation. Where an abnormality is found, to treat the abnormality is much easier than treating hirsutism in an otherwise normal female.

SKIN PROBLEMS

The onset of puberty is associated with a considerable increase in the amount of sebum (grease) that the sebaceous glands produce. This is largely due to the increasing amounts of androgen that are circulating in both sexes at puberty. Boys tend to have greasier skin than girls simply because of their additional (testicular) testosterone secretion. In both sexes, the sebum can readily plug the follicles from which it has been secreted and form what is called a comedo (blackhead) which consists of a reddened conical swelling from which sebum can be expelled. The body surface is covered with bacteria, yeasts and fungi and, unfortunately, whenever body secretions are blocked (urine, bile, cerebrospinal fluid, etc.) they may become infected. When a comedo becomes infected, a pustule appears and may discharge pus.

This problem of spots in the adolescent is extremely common and generally nothing to be very concerned about. The inflammation resolves because the pus discharges and no scarring occurs. If, however, there are many spots or if the infections and the inflammatory response to them are very marked, unsightly cysts and nodular lesions may develop which heal leaving scars. This is not only unsightly at the time but also has distressing long-term consequences.

In the majority of instances, relatively simple measures are effective. These involve keeping the skin, particularly of the face, scrupulously clean with ordinary soap and water and avoiding heavy, especially oily based, make-up creams which serve to exacerbate the problem. This is particularly unwelcome advice for a girl who is trying to conceal her acne by wearing heavy make-up. There are many light foundations, etc., suited to teenage skins on the market which achieve the desired effect.

It has never been satisfactorily explained why acne is particularly a problem of teenagers. Exactly the same endocrinological and skin environment remains in older persons but after the teenage years, acne is a thing of the past for most people. This is presumably why medical means other than the very simple ones outlined above to avoid acne are so manifestly unsatisfactory. As well as topical cleanliness, systemic antibiotics can be taken to reduce infection, but it is really a question of waiting until the condition spontaneously improves.

In patients who have had severe acne, the scarring may be very distressing. In such a situation there are operations which plastic surgeons can undertake to remove the scars of acne. It is certainly worth contemplating such operations if there are serious long-term problems in individual patients.

MENSTRUAL PROBLEMS

The onset of menstrual bleeding is simply a question of the rise and fall of oestrogen secretion and if puberty is otherwise proceeding normally, there is no need to worry about the start of the periods, since they are highly likely to begin. When they fail to do so, it may become necessary to take further steps to ensure that the situation is a normal one. Fortunately, the advent of ultrasound as a method of looking at the ovaries and uterus is an invaluable tool in this respect. It is certainly very important not to induce vaginal bleeding by the administrations of oestrogens without proper investigation. It is almost certain that the majority of girls who have problems establishing regular periods after they stop oestrogen (oral contraceptive) treatment usually had problems before they started the treatment and in fact often only started on the treatment because of those problems. It should be reemphasized that this discussion is simply about a lack of periods with otherwise completely normal puberty. If there is any other abnormality of puberty, failure of breast or pubic hair development, the situation is quite different and requires immediate investigation and management (Chapter 9).

While problems of the failure of the onset of menstrual periods are relatively uncommon, irregular vaginal bleeding (dysfunctional uterine bleeding) is extremely common. It has already been indicated that the first year or two after menarche, uterine bleeding is not generally associated with ovulation and is therefore relatively irregular. If long periods of time elapse between vaginal bleedings, the periods may be heavy and even frightening. The sight of blood is usually much more alarming than the actual amount of blood that is lost. If you doubt this, prick your finger and put a drop of blood into a glass of water. You will be surprised at the effect.

If irregular bleeding becomes a serious problem, it is possible to regulate the periods. This can be done by using some sort of oestrogen medication in a cyclical fashion until normal menstrual cycles have been established when dysfunctional uterine bleeding disappears.

Ovulatory cycles, on the other hand, carry the problem of dysmenorrhoea. This is rarely so severe as to interfere with normal life but when it does so, it can again be completely relieved by suppressing ovulation. Cyclical oestrogen treatment (oral contraceptives) can be used in this situation also but there are, of course, the well-known hazards associated with oral contraception and recourse to this treatment should not be lightly taken.

Finally, the cessation of periods after they have once begun (secondary amenorrhoea) is a much more serious symptom and needs evaluation at an early stage. This is a rare occurrence but periods that have started and then ceased should be investigated, preferably by a specialist in reproductive endocrinology.

INFECTIOUS DISEASES

On the whole, the adolescent years are ones that are relatively free of infections. The common viral infections of childhood, measles, mumps, rubella, chicken pox and so on should have been prevented by immunization. If they were not prevented, they have probably been experienced. Glandular fever, on the other hand, seems to be virtuously synonomous with being an adolescent and it has been called the 'kissing disease'. The infective agent of glandular fever (infectious mononucleosis) is the Epstein—Barr virus. Primary infection with the virus occurs frequently during childhood and provokes insignificant symptoms. Such an infection does, however, confer lifelong immunity to the virus but it does also mean that the virus is intermittently shed from the tissues of the mouth and throat into the saliva. Thus, adolescents who have previously had glandular fever as children can pass it on to other unimmunized adolescents without too much difficulty–hence the 'kissing disease'.

The incubation period of infectious mononucleosis is quite long and there are non-specific symptoms of malaise, lassitude and headache. Sore throats, which can be very painful, and swollen glands may last for a long time. There may also be skin rashes and other more severe systemic symptoms. Investigation of a blood specimen will usually confirm the diagnosis but occasionally the blood test is negative. This is usually because there is another virus which is causing similar symptoms. Cytomegalovirus, for example, may produce an illness which is indistinguishable from glandular fever. Different viral rashes also look extremely similar (which is why the myth that you can get German measles several times has arisen) and it is usually not possible with any certainty to diagnose glandular fever without laboratory tests. These are not usually necessary, because the condition is self-limiting. The problem is that it may take a very long time for the symptoms entirely to disappear. For the most part, they respond to treatment with simple remedies, such as aspirin, but occasionally when they are very severe, stronger remedies may be called for. These, of course, require full medical evaluation.

The other infectious disease which is particularly likely to occur in adolescence is infectious hepatitis. Very much the same considerations apply to this condition as to infectious mononucleosis (glandular fever) or other viral infections. Infectious hepatitis is, however, potentially more serious than the other infections since it can lead to severe liver damage which may be lifelong. Jaundice is a serious symptom and should never be experienced without consulting medical advice.

11

Emotional Problems

There is a widely held belief strongly fostered in prose and poetry that childhood and schooldays are idyllic and the best time of life. This probably reflects the fact that there is a long period of insecurity between childhood and when an adult is settled in a secure situation with satisfactory employment and a happy family life, a goal which many may fail to achieve. The child growing up realizes that real life is not a bed of roses and such realization may be a shock, even in the most secure of family environments. When there are other tensions (marital problems, employment problems for the parents, financial constraints and so on), the growing consciousness of the child to such uncomfortable thoughts not unnaturally produces swings of moods.

It is obvious that people go up and down in their mood and some people go further up and further down than others, which may become so extreme as to constitute a manic-depressive illness, but most people vary from day to day. Adolescent moods may therefore be looked upon as a normal phase of emotional development but they are more obvious than most peoples's mood swings because they are relatively disinhibited. One of the things which humans have to learn in an overcrowded society is to contain the extremes of their emotion so that they can cope with the close proximity of others. When they fail to do so through the disinhibiting effect of, say, alcohol, the result may be very frightening—witness the behaviour of drunken football fans.

Adolescents have also to cope with a large amount of physical energy, with relatively few responsibilities beyond responsibility for themselves and an increasing amount perhaps of leisure time as the working week becomes shortened. For those without employment, the occupation of their time is a considerable social problem for all these reasons.

It is no wonder, therefore, that the adolescent taking his or her place in society experiences swings of mood and reacts to these often in a rather histrionic fashion. The behaviour of the adolescent, as far as others are concerned at this time, appears extremely selfish, boorish and boring. Unfortunately, there does not seem to be any easy solution to such a phase of life: one has to live with the physical changes of childhood and adolescence and one has to put up with the emotional changes as well. It is a regrettable fact that reason plays as small a part in coping with the emotional storms of adolescence as it does in coping with the temper tantrums of the toddler age group. Patience and love on all sides are needed to get through what can seem to be not only an extremely tiresome phase of life but also a very extended one.

With this background, it is hardly surprising that there is a considerable amount of psychiatric disease in adolescence. A classic study of the incidence of psychiatric disorders of children showed a threefold increase in problems of fourteen year olds compared to problems in children aged ten years. A 7 per cent incidence of psychiatric disorder in the latter rose to 21 per cent during adolescence. Furthermore, nearly half of adolescents showed signs of disturbance such as suicidal thoughts, feelings of lack of worth and misery, none of which met the stringent standards necessary for psychiatric diagnosis but which were nevertheless potentially serious. When such behaviour is so very common, it must surely be regarded as part of normal development, but it is still a matter of concern for the adolescents themselves and for their parents and teachers, many of whom may not appreciate the extent of the turmoil being experienced by their children or pupils.

Contrary to general belief, the prognosis of true psychiatric disorder is not better in adolescence than in adults and serious adolescent disturbance should be taken seriously, because skilled professional help given early can prevent a situation from deteriorating.

PSYCHIATRIC PROBLEMS OF ADOLESCENCE

Disorders seen in adolescence may be divided into three groups: those which continue from earlier in childhood, those which are specific to the period of adolescence and psychiatric disorders which mainly occur in adult life but which may have an early onset.

The first group covers behaviour patterns which may be acceptable in smaller children but which cannot be tolerated in older persons. Stealing, lying and truancy can be regarded very differently in a six year old compared to a fourteen year old. Increase in size and emerging sexuality may exacerbate aggressive tendencies, such as bullying, and overflow into violent behaviour which may be seen not only from those who are physically advanced but, particularly, from those who are delayed in their physical maturation and who need to draw attention to themselves by deviant behaviour. The gradually less protected environment of a secondary school may turn occasional school truanting into school refusal and competitive examinations may result in severe anxiety states and other abnormal behaviour patterns. When a parent or child becomes seriously concerned that their behaviour may be getting out of control, reference to a third party, often a doctor, may be very reassuring or may lead to proper professional assistance.

DISORDERS SPECIFIC TO ADOLESCENCE

Where adolescent behaviour deteriorates into juvenile delinquency is a line which is hard to draw, but it is a recurring theme in caring for children that the patterns of behaviour seen in parents are reproduced in their children: thus the major determinants of juvenile deliquency are genetic, family and school influences, all of which tend to be reproduced from generation to generation. Like so much else, the contribution of health professionals is very limited because those who seek help from such professionals are well down the road towards dealing with the problem themselves. It should be the aim of the caring professions, including social workers, teachers and health professionals, to try early to identify parents who are not able to cope with behaviour problems, adolescents who are getting into trouble, and marital disharmony, which is likely to lead to problems for all. Families containing handicapped children are particularly vulnerable in this situation and the early detection of and attention to these problems may assist in preventing extremes of juvenile deliquency.

Depression in adolescents resembles depression in younger children and in adults but is not quite the same as either. In the adult, the classical signs of depression (sleep disturbance, eating disorders, lack of affect, loss of drive and so on) are relatively obvious when they appear in someone who has functioned well until that time. The same is not true in the adolescent in whom these features may appear as a response to many of the demands that are part of the adolescent process. It may be difficult (but it is important) to distinguish between the mood swings of normal adolescents and true depression because active management of the latter will be appropriate whereas the mood swings of normal adolescents have to be endured.

The signs that serious illness may be at hand and that specialist help is required include the following:

(1) sudden academic failure,
(2) isolation from peers,
(3) confusion of fantasy and reality,
(4) behaviour patterns of earlier childhood,
(5) sudden loss of energy,
(6) suicidal ideas,
(7) pain and fatigue,
(8) serious feelings of worthlessness,
(9) changes in appetite and body weight, either increased or decreased.

Attention to these symptoms may enable depression to be diagnosed and treated before it seriously interferes with the ability to function in everyday life and before the depression becomes so oppressive that suicide is considered. Although the suicide rate has fallen in recent years, the incidence of suicide attempts has greatly increased and most of the attempts are by adolescents, usually in the form of a cry for help. Suicide is nevertheless a major cause of death in adolescence: young women frequently attempt suicide but relatively seldom succeed, whereas when a young man attempts suicide, which is less often, he is more likely to succeed.

It is worth briefly considering the factors which make a depressed adolescent attempt suicide. Family turmoil is certainly very important, including the loss of a parent through death or divorce. Family tensions can be increased by parents who either excessively control their children or who reject them. However, it is an acute change which usually precipitates the development of suicidal thoughts and actions. In general, it is a change which occurs in the amount or quality of love, affection, support or respect received by the adolescent from any one of the many sources, peer group, family, friends or others, which form part of the adolescent background.

Most adolescents are aware of having experienced at some time an idea about suicide. Usually such thoughts are suppressed but they may be voiced openly and should not be contemptuously dismissed, although panic reaction is also inappropriate. Whereas adults who declare a suicidal intention often carry it out, adolescents rarely do. Much more dangerous is the adolescent who remarks that 'everything is going to be alright' or 'you won't have to worry about me any more' when there is no reason to believe that things have changed. When serious concerns are raised, the degree of threat can be recognized in the suicidal plan that may have been made. The taking of a mild overdose of sleeping tablets or alcohol is usually an expression of despair or anger; more lethal agents, such as the use of poison or violent actions are much more serious. The site of a suicidal attempt is also important as it tends to indicate the likelihood of discovery before it is too late to reverse the effects of the action.

When an adolescent contemplates suicide, one consideration is often the impact the action will have on others. Sometimes it is seen as an action which will punish families and friends, but at other times it may be used to test whether they 'really care'. Adolescents who seriously contemplate or actually make suicide attempts are frequently saddened or embarrassed by their thoughts and must be given opportunity to express their feelings and talk about them in a receptive setting. Extra care has to be taken with those who are reluctant to discuss their feelings and actions and especially those who appear resentful that their action or intention was discovered before they were able to complete it. Family consultation led by an independent professional is usually the best way to overcome this culminating crisis of severe adolescent depression.

EATING DISORDERS

Excessive eating or refusal to eat are common problems in adolescence. Children discover very early in life that the quickest way to provoke anxiety in their parents, particularly their mothers, is to eat abnormally, especially to refuse food. It is little wonder that in adolescence, one of the goals of which is to establish independence from parents, eating patterns are often a cause for dispute within the family. In general those patterns of eating are not dangerous but both excessive eating and undereating (or excessive eating followed by vomitting or the taking of purgative medicine) can become sufficiently serious to entrain secondary consequences. When this occurs, help is needed.

In medical terms, overeating is the lesser of the two extremes but it may be regarded as a manifestation of very severe unhappiness. Most adolescents are very conscious of the appearance of their bodies and they certainly do not wish to become fat and ugly. When a person abuses himself or herself by becoming excessively obese, the reasons behind such behaviour need careful examination. A morbid fear of obesity may also be a warning sign and avoidance of obesity through excessive physical activity comes into this category.

Although physical activity is frequently altered during adolescence, it is important to realize that the contribution of physical activity to body composition is considerably less than that of food intake. Nevertheless, obese adolescents are observed to be inactive and their inactivity certainly contributes to their obesity. Their obesity equally contributes to their inactivity. The same applies to happiness. Obese people are often unhappy but whether they are fat because they are unhappy or unhappy because they are fat is very difficult to unravel.

What has to be remembered is that changes in body fat do not occur overnight and that alteration of body composition means an alteration of lifestyle and a change of diet over a period of many months. In the context of obesity, it is rare that glandular disorders play a part in the genesis of the condition in adolescence but if there are other abnormalities, such as hirsutism, amenorrhoea, headaches, visual disturbances or an unusual pattern of fat deposition, a medical opinion should be sought.

Anorexia is a potentially more serious disorder, since it can actually lead to death. In an adolescent who is losing weight, it is obviously necessary first to exclude physical disease: anorexia nervosa is concerned with the determined restriction of calorie intake and probably affects about 1 per cent of the adolescent population. The disorder is very much more common in females than in males and tends to have a rather higher incidence among upper social classes. The condition is characterized by a persistent refusal to eat (even though the patient may feel hungry), a distortion of body image so that the patient may think he or she is fat when the very reverse is true. The patient characteristically has boundless physical and mental energy and often has a preoccupation with preparing and administering food to others while denying it to themselves.

The loss of body weight seems to affect normal endocrine function and the characteristic manifestation of this disorder in girls is secondary amenorrhoea. Some believe this to be a manifestation simply of the weight loss: others (like myself) believe that the psychological causes of the lack of appetite also affect the pulsatile secretion of the gonadotrophins. Treatment which enables the patient to gain weight may also enable normal gonadotrophin secretion to be resumed. There is, however, a fairly clear relationship between the state of nutrition and reproductive capability in patients who are not psychiatrically ill (women in prisoner of war camps do not menstruate) but the relationship is certainly complicated and not fully understood.

The management of the disorders of eating is directed towards helping the patient achieve an emotional state where he or she can eat normally. In severe cases it may be necessary to remove the patient from the home environment and such a removal often of itself provokes a crisis which enables behavioural therapy to be successful. A family approach is also required, whether or not the patient is separated from the rest of the family, to try to determine the antecedents of the eating disorder and to correct them.

DRUG ABUSE

Young people commonly experiment with a wide range of easily obtained substances which alter consciousness. These will include tobacco, alcohol, sleeping medicines and volatile solvents such as glue. Experimenting with these substances may be regarded as a normal part of growing up but experiments with amphetamines, barbiturates, cocaine, heroin, LSD and other illicit drugs verge on the deliquent. Unfortunately, adults may either collude in encouraging such experimentation or may profit from it. Whether cannabis (hash, marihuana) is more or less harmful than tobacco or alcohol is not the point here. The fact is that at present it is an illegal drug and obtaining it brings an adolescent into contact with unscrupulous providers who would be more than happy to convert the occasional taker of cannabis into the regular customer for heroin.

Stories of adolescents becoming addicted to drugs and then entering a life of crime or prostitution to pay for them are too common to require rehearsing here. It needs only to be said that society has a duty to protect adolescents against exploitation of this type and the normal adolescent needs no more to experiment with drug taking than does a surgeon need to suffer the condition for which regularly he performs an operation. Psychotherapeutic help to the individual who has drug problems and to the family is urgently needed and should be rapidly mobilized for those in whom drug taking appears to be becoming a problem.

THE EARLY ONSET OF ADULT PSYCHIATRIC DISORDERS

Both the major psychoses, schizophrenia and manic depressive psychosis, may present in adolescence. Schizophrenia is an extremely serious handicapping mental illness which needs to be recognized and treated as soon as possible. The schizophrenic appears to be depressed (lack of affect) but also manifests changes of thought, which does not proceed logically and may be associated with the use of curious language, of feelings, which may involve acute persecution complexes, and of perception, the seeing of visions and the hearing of voices. These symptoms should be regarded very seriously and referred to an expert as soon as possible.

Manic-depressive psychosis is less common in adolescence. The depressive component is relatively easy to spot but the manic phase is often more disabling in terms of the ability to work and to cope with everyday life. Very rapid swings may occur from depression to mania and the reverse, and these swings may account for apparently inexplicable suicides during adolescence. Because of the risk of suicide, an adolescent experiencing extreme swings of mood should be referred to a psychiatrist for diagnosis and management.

Neurotic disorders seen in adult life, such as depression, anxiety, obsessional behaviour and phobias, are commonly present in adolescence. Physically handicapped adolescents are particularly vulnerable to neurotic disturbance, presumably because they become faced with the realities of their limitations which can cause profound psychiatric disorders. This is an area par excellence where preventive counselling may be of assistance.

Adult-type depression should be relatively easy to recognize in the adolescent and responds well to treatment. It is not as commonly associated with suicidal behaviour as true adolescent depression discussed above.

Anxiety is a natural and necessary part of functioning in adult life. Adolescent anxieties about the future must, therefore, be regarded as realistic and within the normal spectrum. Nevertheless, they can assume a disproportionate feature of life that prevents normal activity and in such an instance, treatment is undoubtedly required.

More serious are anxieties about sexual performance. Homosexual anxieties are common in boys during adolescence and indeed homosexual experimentation may be regarded as part of normal adolescence. It is estimated that about 10 per cent of men have a permanent homosexual orientation and considerable care has therefore to be taken about the counselling of adolescents who are worried about their sexuality. Girls are less frequently affected by homosexual anxieties, although this may change with the increasing publicity given to lesbianism. It is usually the parents of adolescents with homosexual tendencies who are more anxious than the adolescents themselves.

The onset of sexual perversions (fetishism, transvestism and sado-masochism) occurs during adolescence. The management of these disorders needs very skilled help which should be sought early in order to enable normal sexual development to occur.

Phobias are the commonest neurotic disorder in adolescence and are usually manifest as school refusal. The presentation to the doctor may often be with somatic symptoms of anxiety (palpitation, headache, abdominal pain, etc.) which are only present on school days. The problem is commonly mismanaged by an excessive preoccupation with the somatic symptoms without understanding the underlying emotional disorder. It is important to get on and to treat the patient rather than to allow the situation to become chronic, when intervention becomes very much more difficult. This is also the case with obsessional neurotic tendencies; these are characterized by compulsive thoughts such as a preoccupation with cleanliness and repetitive actions such as handwashing which are unwelcome but which cannot be resisted. Sometimes they mask the onset of schizophrenia but this is usually not the case. Early treatment is required to try to prevent obsessional neurotic tendencies before they become chronic and intractable.

MANAGEMENT AND TREATMENT OF PSYCHIATRIC DISORDERS

Adolescents provoke, even in professional people, anger, irritation, envy and even sexual arousement and adolescents are often very sensitive to the moods which they can provoke in adults. Treatment of mental disorder in adolescence is, therefore, a very specialized field which needs to be undertaken by those who are specially trained to cope with their own feelings, which does not apply to every medical practitioner. Access to a child or adolescent psychiatrist may not be very easy because of the number of adolescents who have problems and the relative paucity of specialists in adolescent psychiatry who necessarily have to deal with the very seriously ill. Thus, many family doctors have become extremely skilled in the handling of the commoner disorders of adolescence and in the counselling of parents of children with the more severe disorders which are treated by adolescent psychiatrists. The family doctor has the major advantage in that he will know what is currently 'normal' within the population for which he cares. He will be in a good position to advise whether the problem is simply one of containment or whether specialist treatment is needed.

12

Sexual Problems

The question of contraception has been considered previously (page 67) but the sexually active adolescent faces additional problems to the main one which will be pregnancy. These include sexually transmitted diseases and disorders of the genital tract associated with sexual activity. For boys, a discharge from the urethra, pain on passing urine or blood in the urine are all symptoms which demand early attention. For girls, irregularity in the menstrual periods, either more frequent bleeding or amenorrhoea, profuse vaginal discharge or urinary symptoms are pointers to venereal disease.

SEXUALLY TRANSMITTED DISEASES

Infections caused by *Haemophilus vaginalis*, *Candida albicans* (monilia), *Trichomonas vaginalis*, *Neisseria gonorrhoeae*, *Chlamydia trachomatis* and *Herpes simplex* can all be transmitted through sexual intercourse. In addition, there is strong evidence that infectious mononucleosis (glandular fever), infectious hepatitis (jaundice) and the acquired immunity deficiency syndrome (AIDS) are all infections which are transmitted by the transfer of infected body secretions. The chances of contracting one of these diseases are greatly increased if the number of sexual partners is increased. This can be simply the result of promiscuous sexual activity (particularly common amongst homosexual men) or of consorting with a partner who is promiscuous. It is important to realize that sexually transmitted diseases may be present in a person, particularly a girl, without causing any symptoms.

Vaginal discharge is a part of normal development in puberty. The reason for this is that the vaginal mucosa changes its character as puberty advances; it becomes thicker and its glycogen content increases. Oestrogen stimulates the production of mucus and the acidity of the vagina increases. The low pH in the vagina may exert a protective effect against various vaginal pathogens but it is fairly obvious when a physiological vaginal discharge becomes a pathological one because the normal vaginal secretions are white or mucoid and the mucus contains small white flecks. A pathological discharge is profuse and uniform in character.

When a vaginal discharge occurs, the only way to make a diagnosis is to take a specimen and to examine it in the laboratory to make a diagnosis of the causative infecting organism. Treatment is based upon this diagnosis and it is important that treatment should also be extended to the sexual partner(s). If the patient does not improve rapidly, she will need to be examined carefully in case there is a foreign body in the vagina. Infection will not clear up until the foreign body is removed.

Some of these infections, notably gonorrhoea, can cause more generalized illness and this is why treatment is so very important. Early recognition of symptoms, immediate investigation and treatment are the keys to a successful outcome.

NEOPLASTIC DISEASE

Cancer of the genital tract is very rare in the teenage population but it is certainly true that the age at which intercourse first occurs and the number of sexual partners both have a significant influence on the incidence of carcinoma of the cervix. The presentation of this condition is usually with a bloody or brown vaginal discharge and this reemphasizes the point that was made previously that such discharges should not be ignored.

PREGNANCY IN ADOLESCENCE

In 1981 in England and Wales 5,330 babies were born to girls of sixteen years of age or less. Schoolgirl pregnancy is generally to the disadvantage of the mother, the infant, their families and society in general. Marriage is rarely a solution for most of the problems of the pregnant schoolgirl and may actually compound her difficulties. The mortality rates for infants of teenage mothers compare unfavourably with those of the offspring of older mothers, excluding mothers aged thirty-five and older. This is partly because teenage mothers are at greater risk of giving birth prematurely but also because there is a considerable increase in the incidence of sudden infant (cot) death.

On the other hand, it is certainly perfectly possible for a teenage mother to bear and rear a child who is perfectly healthy in every way, but such a mother needs a considerable amount of support in doing so.

It is wrong to suppose that most teenage pregnancies arise from promiscuous behaviour. Teenage pregnancies generally arise from fairly stable relationships and may indeed even have been consciously planned in some instances. They may occasionally arise as a result of a single act of sexual intercourse, but this is not usually the case.

The problem for many teenage mothers is that they often come from rather deprived backgrounds and becoming a teenage mother does little for establishing themselves in better circumstances. It gives little confidence for the future of the baby if he or she stays with the mother: if the baby is given in adoption, the care that adopting parents will give is likely to be of high quality, but the emotional consequences for the mother giving away her baby are considerable and the plight of the teenage mother is a sad one. Given the ready availability of effective methods of contraception, it is important to encourage adolescents wishing to experiment with sexual relationships to take advantage of such methods.

Practical Advice

If a teenager does become pregnant, it is important early to consult a doctor. One of the problems of the pregnancies of teenage mothers is that attendance at antenatal clinics is very poor and this is a potential hazard to the baby. Further, if the mother were to wish to consider the alternative of abortion, the earlier she starts making the arrangements the better it is for all concerned. One reason for delay is often the hope that the pregnancy will spontaneously miscarry. Although about 10 per cent of pregnancies do miscarry, this is not a wise course. Doctors are used to being involved in these situations and, whatever the patient may feel, the doctor will certainly not be embarrassed.

In this connection it must be remembered that some adolescents may not actually recognize the symptoms of pregnancy or may deny the possibility of being pregnant. Consequently pregnancy may present to health professionals with many different symptoms. Morning nausea with or without vomiting, increased appetite and increasing tenderness of the breasts may be unassociated in the mind of an adolescent with her secondary amenorrhoea. Weight gain is a complaint with which some adolescents present but weight loss can also be a feature of early pregnancy. Other more vague symptoms may be present such as pain, which may not necessarily be localized to the abdomen, fatigue and the weight loss which may follow morning sickness or attempts to conceal the fact that one is pregnant. Occasionally an adolescent just asks for a check-up and a request for this with a degree of urgency should alert the possibility of the adolescent being pregnant.

Antenatal care is important for teenage mothers because they have a rather high incidence of toxaemia (high blood pressure and fluid retention) which is dangerous for the baby. They may often have long taken a diet which is rather poor in iron content and severe anaemia of pregnancy is not uncommonly seen in pregnant adolescents. The actual delivery of the baby is usually not a problem for the adolescent, rather less indeed than for the older mother, but the incidence of breast feeding, attendance at infant welfare clinics and rates of immunization of the baby are all strikingly decreased in adolescent mothers. The conduct of pregnancy and childbirth in the adolescent is therefore very demanding (and sometimes very frustrating) for health professionals, but in view of the problems that they face, teenage mothers deserve all the sympathy and help that they can get.

13

Skeletal Problems

Adolescents are susceptible to the bone and joint problems which afflict adults and children but they are also liable to problems which have their origin at the time of adolescence, not least because this is a time of considerable physical energy and traumatic lesions are certainly the most common of those seen.

Trauma can lead to sprains, strains and fractures. Fortunately adolescents heal quickly and simple remedies are all that are needed for the majority of such injuries. Some conditions associated with trauma are more difficult to treat and Osgood-Schlatter disease, which affects the insertion of the patellar (knee cap) tendon into the tibia, is one such disease. It usually affects boys between the ages of ten and fifteen and especially the sporting enthusiast. Pain over the front of the top of the shin is aggravated by exertion and there is local tenderness. The problem is that although the condition resolves spontaneously, it may take as long as a year to get better.

The laxity of ligaments, which is characteristic of children and may be seen in some adolescents, may be a considerable advantage in sporting prowess. It is, however, important to take care of joints which have extreme mobility because they are easily damaged and repeated damage to joints brings on premature osteoarthritis. Supple joints are highly prized but the progressive stretching of ligaments is not good for joint stability—aerobics may therefore have long-term consequences.

DISORDERS OF THE HIP

Pain in the hip should always be taken seriously but it is important to remember that the pain which originates in the hip may often be felt in the knee. Pain which is severe enough to cause a limp should always be investigated. While traumatic and infective causes will be high on the list, there are three conditions which occur in young persons which deserve especial mention.

The first, which usually presents in very early childhood, is congenital dislocation of the hip. In this condition the cup (acetabulum) which the head of the femur forms in the pelvic girdle during foetal life fails to form and the hip joint is thus unstable. If this is missed in infancy, the consequences may be serious and, by the time of adolescence, arthritis can already have begun.

The second condition, which presents in the slightly older school child is Perthe's disease. In this condition the articulating part of the head of the femur, the epiphysis, becomes soft, irregular and flattened. Thus it does not articulate properly with the acetabulum which causes pain and limb shortening. By the time of adolescence, this has generally subsided and healed but occasionally very severe cases, which may have become static in later childhood, begin to cause problems in adolescence with arthritis. Skilled advice about what to do is urgently needed.

Finally, a condition which occurs especially in adolescents is slippage of the upper femoral epiphyses. When this occurs, the cartilagenous plate between the femoral shaft and its epiphysis, which articulates with the acetabulum to form the hip joint, fractures allowing the epiphysis to slip which causes pain and a limp. The weakness of the plate is believed to be caused by an imbalance between growth hormone and sex hormones and it certainly occurs particularly in children who have endocrine disorders. A precipitating traumatic event seems to be quite common in this condition for which surgical treatment is generally recommended.

SCOLIOSIS

Scoliosis consists of two elements, a lateral spinal curvature and also a rotational abnormality. The latter may present as distortion of the chest wall. Scoliosis is not generally a condition associated with pain.

There are two main groups of patients with scoliosis. The first comprises those in whom the deformity is mobile and can be fully corrected, either actively or passively. In these patients, the deformity does not progress and may disappear spontaneously or when an underlying cause is removed. Such a cause may be postural, especially in the tall adolescent, may be compensatory if one leg is shorter than the other, as it may often be in a child who was born of low birthweight, and it may be secondary to a spinal lesion, the adolescent leaning to one side to relieve the pressure on nerve roots.

The second type of scoliosis is rigid and cannot be easily corrected either actively or passively. Patients with these curves have a progressive deformity which needs attention. Unfortunately, for the majority of patients, the cause of this type of scoliosis is not known. Idiopathic scoliosis may have its onset at any age during growth but most commonly presents during periods of extremely rapid growth, such as in early infancy or in adolescence. There is a curious sex difference in that boys are most commonly affected by infantile idiopathic scoliosis, whereas girls tend to develop adolescent scoliosis and they tend to be tall and thin. In rare instances, scoliosis may result from vertebral abnormalities and from any one of a very large number of neurological problems. Since the key to management is early recognition of the curve, early referral to a specialist in scoliosis (and not all orthopaedic surgeons are expert in scoliosis) should result in the rapid diagnosis of a possible cause of scoliosis. Scoliosis in a child who is growing very rapidly needs especial attention.

Once the curve has been detected and classified, a careful check must be made to ensure that it does not become progressively worse. This depends upon the assessment of skeletal radiographs and intervention is required if the degree of curve increases significantly. If observation suggests that the curve is deteriorating, the first treatment will be external splinting in the form of a brace with possible resort to surgical correction if this is not effective. Hitherto rather little work has been done about possible managements of scoliosis by medical means, but since scoliosis is associated with the rapid growth of adolescents, it should in future be possible to adjust the rate of growth, particularly in a tall individual, to the benefit of the orthopaedic condition.

OTHER ACHES AND PAINS IN ADOLESCENCE

Pain in the back may arise from vertebral problems and should be taken seriously. It can be a symptom of malignant disease. It can also occur in association with inflammatory bowel disease, psoriasis and other skin disorders. Ankylosing spondylitis is also an important cause of back pain which has three separate components. The spondylitis (inflammation of the vertical joints) which is characteristically associated with morning stiffness and relieved by exercise and made worse by rest responds to treatment with anti-inflammatory drugs, such as aspirin, and exercises. The sacrolitis (inflammation of the joints between the spine and pelvic girdle) is an extension of the spondylitis but the third component, peripheral polyarthritis, is often missed and thought to be part of another generalized arthritis, such as Still's disease. Still's disease is a different condition since it has manifestations and problems in many body systems, not just the joints.

All these conditions sound rather frightening but it must be remembered that they are rather rare whereas aches and pains in adolescence, sometimes called growing pains, which are not serious are very common. Most adolescents with pains do not have serious disorders but since early recognition and treatment of serious skeletal disorders can prevent long-term consequences, aches and pains need certainly to be taken seriously in the first instance. A thorough physical examination by an experienced doctor will reveal whether aches and pains are likely to be of significance.

14

Extremes of Size

Adolescents are generally very occupied with their bodies, often rightly, since they are of considerable attraction. Attention to complexion and hair occupies a considerable amount of time, to the benefit of the cosmetic trade. The corollary of this attention is that for those whose bodies fall outside the normal ranges, great unhappiness can ensue. This may apply to being short, being tall, being fat, being thin and being excessively delayed in sexual development. Precocious sexual development, which is a cause of great anxiety to parents, does not seem greatly to bother most of the patients themselves.

SHORT STATURE AND DELAYED PUBERTY

The commonest cause for being short during adolescence is that the whole process of growth is extended so that the delay in growth leads to the adolescent being left behind by his or her peers both in terms of size and sexual development. This can be a cause of great unhappiness and as it is often remediable, it is well worth seeking assistance. This may be given in the form of help for growth alone or help for growth and sexual maturation, since the latter cannot be achieved without some increase in height. The problems of patients who have isolated delay in sexual maturation have been covered on page 83.

Short stature generally divides itself into two main groups: people who are short with normal body proportions and look normal and people who have varieties of skeletal disorder, which are manifested by differential shortening of the arms and legs compared to the spine. Occasionally the abnormality predominantly affects the spine. While height is a strongly genetically determined condition, it is important not to dismiss the short child of short parents without careful thought, since what may have not been treatable in the parents may now be treatable in their children.

Classical teaching indicates that treatment is only available for short children who are growing slowly and in general terms this is certainly true. There is, however, increasing interest and attention being focused upon the various treatments which may become available for the adjustment of normal stature which may be highly desirable for social purposes. A talented ballet dancer with a height prediction of 5ft 1in may well be denied access to the corps de ballet for which the minimum height qualification is 5ft 2in. It may be possible in coming years to attain an extra inch in such circumstances through the administration of extra growth hormone or through other manipulation of growth hormone secretion by pharmacological means. At present this is not a realizable prospect but it is likely to become so within the decade.

For children who look normal but are not growing normally, a diagnosis and treatment is urgently required. This should have been introduced before adolescence but occasionally it is the failure of sexual maturation in association with short stature which particularly draws attention to a problem. As already indicated, in boys this is most likely due to simple delay of puberty but in girls, although simple delay does occur, it is very important to be assured that ovarian function is normal and that the patient is not suffering from gonadal dysgenesis.

Many patients with short stature lack confidence during

adolescence and come to undervalue themselves. This may lead them to perform badly in examinations and it is most important that short adolescents receive sympathy, understanding and help, even if they do not actually receive medical treatment. There are, however, increasing things which can be done to improve growth of small adolescents and this must be greatly welcomed for their long-term happiness.

TALL STATURE

Tall stature is a considerable advantage during the early school years, at least for the child who is able to cope with being treated as older than he or she actually is. Sometimes, being treated as a child considerably older leads to the child wishing to make clear that he or she is not as old as all that and the child may then develop regressive symptoms to make such a demonstration. Generally speaking, however, the tall child is at an educational advantage which may cease to be the case during adolescence. Most tall children tend to go into puberty early and thus bring their growth to its natural end early without remaining excessively tall. In these patients, the change from being one of the tallest at school to being of average or even of small height may come as something of a shock. For children who do not go early into puberty the continuation of growth can lead to excessively tall stature and very considerable problems in adult life. These are generally worse for girls than for boys, presumably because girls are generally smaller than boys and being out of the ordinary causes problems.

Trying to do something about an excessively tall height prediction requires adjustment of growth rate and sometimes alteration in the timing of the onset of puberty. The earlier a patient presents to a physician who specializes in this area, therefore, the better it is and the easier are the prospects to adjust final height. One of the saddest experiences is to encounter a patient who has already become extremely tall who wishes that they were not in that position but for whom the time in which adjustment could be made has already passed.

The methods of adjusting final height have until now largely involved induction of early puberty and causing a rapid advance of skeletal maturation by the administration of large doses of sex steroids. Since such treatments are unphysiological and involve large doses of medication, alternative methods are currently a matter of considerable interest. There may be pharmacological ways of slowing down growth which are safer than the manipulation of puberty, although it must be stressed that many thousands of children have had tall stature presented by the manipulation of puberty and no harm has yet been reported from any one of them.

DISPROPORTIONATE GROWTH

For adolescents who have tall or short stature which is associated with abnormalities of limb growth or trunk growth, either diminished or increased, it is important to make a diagnosis of the condition, even if it is a familial one. There are a number of specific complications which are associated with disproportionate growth, many of which can be avoided by early recognition and careful management. The diagnosis of conditions involving disproportionate growth is not very easy and requires the skills of physicians and particularly of radiologists which are acquired by only a very few. Referral to a centre for the assessment of growth disorders is highly desirable for such patients. The average district general hospital does not have sufficient experience in the diagnosis and management of these disorders simply because they do not see enough of them.

OBESITY

Obesity means the excessive accumulation of subcutaneous fat and this can only be acquired through the consumption of food in excess of normal energy requirements. Conversely, it can only be lost by restriction of energy intake (see page 52).

In general, an excessive intake of calories leads to tall stature in early life and most obese adolescents are tall for their age. In such a situation they are very unlikely to have any form of glandular disorder. For the adolescent or child who is not growing normally, however, this is not the case and obesity which is associated with short stature should be investigated early, since it may be due to a relatively easily treatable endocrine disorder. It may also be the symptom of a disorder which carries serious consequences in later life, such as Cushing syndrome, which if treated early may be curable without any long-term problems.

Obesity may also be associated with mental handicap. A simple rule can therefore be applied to those who are afflicted with obesity. If they are of normal size and have normal sexual development, the remedy is in their own hands. For those who are short or mentally retarded or both, referral to a physician to exclude other disorders is very desirable. Even if a primary condition cannot be discovered, the secondary consequences of excessive obesity can often be helped.

THINNESS

Most patients who are thin do not have anything wrong with them but the medical causes of loss of weight are serious and a sudden change in body size requires an explanation, even if that explanation is entirely benign. In particular, in girls the problem of anorexia nervosa may be far from obvious even to very near relatives and the consequences of this condition (page 116) are sufficiently serious that early treatment is certainly indicated.

15

Other Serious Medical Disorders

The treatment and management of disease in adolescents rarely differs from treatment at other times of life but the complex emotional situation in which an adolescent exists may considerably alter both the course of the disorder and the reactions of those around them.

A typical example may be found in diabetes mellitus. This is a condition which is common and which is relatively easy to treat. All that is needed is to match the insulin administered to the insulin deficient patient with the food that he or she is going to eat and to make adjustments for the energy which will be expended in exercise so that the condition, relatively speaking, takes care of itself. Such a mechanistic explanation, although it is actually true, is very far from reality.

In normal persons, the taking of food is associated with a rise in blood sugar and a consequent secretion of insulin into the blood which passes to the liver. This enables the blood sugar to be rapidly adjusted to within normal limits over a very short time and within very fine boundaries. In the diabetic, insulin is given before the meal is taken. It is given not into the circulation which leads directly to the liver but into a part of the body in which insulin is rarely found in any large amount. Since insulin is given before eating, rather than rising afterwards, the dose that is given is estimated on the basis of what the diabetic expects (or is expected) to eat and the consequence is that the diabetic has to eat exactly the same at exactly the same time every single day if a normal stable blood sugar level is to be achieved. It is little wonder that it is so difficult to control the blood sugar of even the most compliant of diabetic patients.

When adolescence comes to a diabetic patient, the situation can become extremely complicated. The parents, who have been responsible for the management of diabetes during childhood, have to start handing over responsibility for diabetic control to their teenage child. When the child is seen to be abusing his or her diabetes and allowing the blood sugar to become excessively high or excessively low, the parent, who may be well aware of the long and short-term dangers of such swings, may become increasingly anxious and may seek to interfere with the management of their child's diabetes. Such a situation inevitably brings conflict and unhappiness, not to mention a deterioration in the quality of diabetic control. The problem can rapidly escalate and the adolescent may demonstrate all sorts of deviant behaviour in order to declare independence of parental restrictions. This leads to school refusal, to manipulating admission to hospital and to other subterfuges to get out of the intolerable situation.

There can be no easy answer to this sort of problem. In a sense, the parents are both right and responsible if they take a continuing interest in their child's diabetic control; on the other hand, to be overly involved in the body of an adolescent wishing to achieve independence is extremely hazardous.

The same problem can be found within the provision of medical care. Paediatric departments in hospitals are generally set up to provide a very friendly service and intimate relationship between the doctors, nurses, parents and children. While a rather similar feeling is engendered in a geriatric unit, hospital services for patients between these two age groups are much more of a 'take it or leave it' variety. The doctor says that this is the treatment (which he may or may not take the trouble to explain) and it is up to the patient whether he or she accepts it. At the extremes of life, considerable effort is devoted into persuading patients to accept treatments which are for their own good. The transition, therefore, for the adolescent from the cosy family atmosphere of a paediatric department to the chilly adult world can be a considerable shock. Wise physicians are taking some steps to ensure a smooth transition of care but it is rarely a period without event.

What applies to diabetes is the quintessence of the problems of providing health care to adolescents with serious disease. Fortunately, cancer, leukaemia and other malignant disorders are relatively rare in adolescence, but when they do arise, just the same problems of doctor–parent–patient relationships arise. Thus, the patient who may be dying of secondary malignant disease may either consciously or unconsciously wound his parents by actively preferring to be in the security of a hospital, where the staff are relatively unemotional about the delivery of care and the nature of his disease, rather than be at home where it is difficult for him to spend the latter days of his life under anything which approaches normal circumstances.

The management of pain in such situations is often used as a pretext for requiring hospital admission and it is a familiar experience that pain which is adequately controlled with relatively simple analgesia within the hospital situation becomes unsupportable at home away from recourse to immediate help. Most people recognize the luxury of surrendering to an illness and its treatment, if only in remembering what it is like to wake up feeling ill and then to discover that the thermometer indicates that one has a raised temperature and is therefore licensed to go back to bed until one feels better! One can feel just as ill and have no signs of illness and thus feel impelled to carry on. In a very small way, this reflects the security which the seriously ill adolescent achieves from surrendering to the care of a hospital rather than fighting his disorder at home with all the complicating emotional circumstances which necessarily surround him there.

Finally, in a chapter devoted to the adolescent with serious medical disease, thought must be given to the other children within a family. It is natural and indeed right that a child or adolescent with a serious disease should be the primary focus of attention while such disease is being diagnosed and treated, but if treatment is going to go on for a long time, an excessive involvement of the family in one particular individual can lead to a break-up of the whole family unit. Husbands and wives need to remember that they have to care for their own relationship, even while dealing with their children's problems. If they fail to cherish that relationship, they may be in danger of finding that when the child's problem has resolved for better or for worse, they have no relationship to which to return. Other children in the family also require support and can become extremely isolated and resentful if all the attention is focused on one member of the family to the exclusion of all others. Serious disease in an adolescent does involve the whole family but should not so dominate the family that all decisions are made with respect to the illness and without due consideration being given to other requirements.

Useful Addresses

Family doctors are in the best position to know where to seek help locally for the majority of problems of adolescence.

Other sources of information:

(1) On problems of growth:
>   Child Growth Foundation
>   2 Mayfield Avenue
>   London W4
>   (01) 995–0257

(2) On drug abuse:
>   (a) The local Citizens' Advice Bureau can help.
>
>   (b) The Standing Conference on Drug Abuse maintains a list of local facilities.
>   1–4 Hatton Place
>   London EC1
>   (01) 431–2341
>
>   (c) A chain of self-help groups also exists and may be contacted through
>   Families Anonymous
>   88 Caledonian Road
>   London N7
>   (01) 278–8805

(3) On sexual problems:

Any family planning clinic will know what local facilities are best.

Index

152